Nursing Nurses

Uncovering the Critical Issues Facing the Heart & Minds of Healthcare

Dr. Sandra Risoldi MSN Ed., DNP, RN, CLNC

This book is dedicated to Nurses, Nursing Assistants and All those that have stood by me throughout this movement…we are only getting started.

Nurses Against Violence Unite, Inc.™

This is about Us.

"I attribute my success to this: I Never gave or took an excuse" ~Florence Nightingale

Introduction

When life throws you lemons you need to make lemonade. We have as a profession have suffered many years of abuse, many times the not, we are told that our opinions do not matter, despite proof of the patient on nurse attack or vengeance from a co-worker, even from upper management. We have been told that nothing is going to change, no matter how much we report things, it will always stay the same. With the rise of nurses leaving the profession in record numbers either continuing their education, disabled due to their jobs, blacklisted for speaking up, the facts speak for themselves. Low job satisfaction scores, high turnover, insufficient nursing education and high acuity, people wonder why there is a "shortage of nurses", it isn't just because we need more. Store greeters at a department stores do not get this abuse, why should we? When founding Nurses Against Violence Unite, Inc.™ it not only give others a voice to speak up about being retaliated against, injured, or made to feel they are inadequate with their care, it allows over 7,000 members to speak up about what is happening to them either on an anonymous platform or we tell their story for them. The guiding force behind the organization is the mission statement to bring awareness, educate, empower other and eliminate violence in the workplace. The contents of this book, is only a portion that has guided the creation of my DNP project but a good indicator of the direction of the innovation that we are bringing the nursing profession and the creation of the first prevention program created by a nurse, for nurses, all healthcare professionals, and beyond. Please Join Us: Facebook.com/groups/NAVUnite

If you are working on a DNP project, ask us how we can assist you with this topic!

Chapter 1

The Beginning

Over the past few years working in a clinical setting, both as a staff member and a clinical instructor, there have been many observed patient incidents involving escalation. The National Database of Nursing Quality Indicators (NDNQI), made it clear, that "psychiatric, physical assault, voluntary nurse turnover, nursing hours per patient day, and RN education" all were related to a shortlist of issues like short staffing (Montalvo, 2007, p. 3). Why would nurses leave their jobs, state openly that they get hit and yelled at by both patient and family members, call off from work that leads to short staffing and eventual turnover? Nurses are not equipped with specific skills and knowledge of working with those that are suffering from severe mental illness or addiction. Due to the high levels of stress, nurses are leaving their facility by either increasing their skills seeking higher education, moving to another facility or leaving nursing altogether (Laeeque, Bilal, Babar, Khan, & Rahman, 2017).

Mental illness is everywhere in a healthcare setting from medical-surgical to mother and baby. For example, purposes, what happens when nurses are not prepared to care for an open-heart post-op patient and have a medical-surgical background? They are advised by the nurse practice act not to take the patient as they, being the trained nursing professional, are not equipped with the knowledge.
Take it another step farther and envision the nurse's stress level when they have no choice and given the patient anyway. The same thing happens when you take the same medical-surgical nurse that is working with acute mental health or an addiction patient. Yes, nurses know basic

health assessment skills but unprepared to adequately care for this population in the capacity of knowing what subjective is real or not, as the person looks okay. Still, the nurse thinks that the patient acts, talks, and is acting rationale. Per the Florida Nurse Practice Act, "failing to meet minimal standards of acceptable and prevailing nursing practice, include engaging in acts for which the nurse is not qualified with training or experience," can lead to disciplinary action (Nurse Practice Act, 2018). If the healthcare system does not account for or put the nurse in a conducive environment to their expertise or knowledge, the nurse will automatically become stressed and sometimes even overloaded if nurses are not working according to their training. When the nurse that is unprepared with adequate baseline mental health and addiction training, as it lacks discipline-wide, it could lead to a near-miss, behavior escalation, or injury to the nurse. Sufficient resources from their employer, from the lack of support, which subsequently falls back onto the nurse, for putting themselves in that situation, ultimately leading to burn-out and post-traumatic stress disorder. The goal is to help nurses stay safe when working with invisible illnesses and be mindful of our own verbal but non-verbal communication. This research was not set to belittle or show signs of weakness in the character of my fellow nurses and nursing staff, but to identify, bring awareness, educate, empower, eliminate violence in the workplace.

When considering a theory that closely correlates with behavior modification, it would be the social cognitive theory that focuses on "continuous, bidirectional interaction of people and their environments, which the resulting behavior affects their environment" (Hodges & Videto, 2011, p. 149). The stressed-out nurse that has not received adequate training to work with severely mentally ill or addicted patients may not respond to a patient in the manner which is conducive to a positive outcome. As a result, the patient's behavior has mirrored the nurse in many situations, resulting in patient escalation. There would be times that the nurse would say appropriate things. Still, their actions would point to not caring, such as adverse facial expressions like eye-rolling, not smiling, poor eye contact, staring at their phone, charting while the patient is talking, or not coming by when telling the patient that they would. Other times, the nurse would be curt, direct, have an elevated tone, and ignore the patient altogether, sending the tech in to see the patient. As the behavior we put out, there can project onto this vulnerable patient and mirror itself back to the nurse.

    Does that nurse mean to portray negative non-verbal communication? By the nurse not having a background in nursing or not understanding the never-ending tasks that we face, it is not entirely their fault. Instead, the result is a product of a failed system with the outcome of exhaustion and feeling helpless no matter which way you turn. Your care will never be the way we hoped when leaving nursing school. Patients pick up on something being wrong and react in a manner that will get a reaction as they do not understand, nor should they have too. When stress plays a role in the delivery of care, it can, directly and indirectly, create an unhealthy situation for not only the patient but also the staff caring for that patient. The goal of this practicum project is to identify the behavior and help nurses to help themselves when it comes to working with acute mental illness and addiction, plus have resources to help them cope, succeed, and feel supported throughout their career.

Planning the Learning Objectives

With the rise of burn-out and post-traumatic stress disorder among nurses, the focus of this practicum project blends the need for increased awareness of verbal and physical communication when working with those with mild to acute mental illness and addiction. In April 2018, the American Nurses Association conducted a poll asking nurses about their experiences with patient on nurse violence. As a result, nurses reported 62 percent, who had been verbally and physically abused by patients (American Nurses Association [ANA], 2018, para. 3). When the nurse is aware of their actions, they can begin to modify their approach to stressful situations and behaviors exhibited by the patient, preventing verbal and physical attacks. The rationale of looking at patient on nurse abuse from this angle stems from the minimal amount of mental health education that is presented in the nursing school curriculum. Consequently, as a result, the nurse is not adequately prepared to care for every patient, both from a mental and physical standpoint, if the patient should become physically abusive.

Recognizing poor communication techniques can be the result of minimal mental health education in nursing; this would be the first step in Bloom's Taxonomy (Armstrong, 2017). In correlation with the number of nurses that are verbally and physically attacked, there may be a direct link to the decrease of self-awareness from the nurse on their actions and behavior regulation. Interpreting this information would be useful for reflecting on one's reactions to the patient's action or verbal outbursts. By implementing an education plan for nurses, a couple of simple techniques could be incorporated to reduce outbursts and violent attacks. With every patient, anticipate needs, set boundaries, keep to your word about timeframes while remaining empathetic, and consistent with the patient's care. The goal is to stay the same way with every patient, thereby reducing burnout and post-traumatic stress disorder for the nurse. The nurse can still be friendly, empathetic, and caring; however, limits should be set according to how much the patient is struggling with their addiction or acute mental illness. Combining the information about how it is possible that the nurse did not have much exposure to critical mental health or addiction, and it could inadvertently trigger the behavior escalation of the patient.

The goal is to combine the updated information by interpreting an innovative way to care for every patient, ranging from mental illness to various medical issues. By creating a teaching plan, it will help the nurse learner to recognize their behavior and nonverbal communication by using scenarios and possible triggers that may produce a negative outcome.

    Aligning the practicum topic to the Doctor of Nursing Practice (DNP) Essentials, it would fall under number one, which is noted as the "scientific underpinnings for practice" as it is "patterning human behavior and interaction with the environment in normal and critical life situations" (American Association of Colleges of Nursing [AACN], 2006, p. 9). By recognizing the potential problem of poor communication techniques, the nurse learner can use self-reflection to help them cope and create a safe environment for both the patient and all staff members. As a result, it could decrease burnout and post-traumatic stress disorder, which could be a contributor to staffing challenges and nursing turnover.

"I've learned that people will forget what you said, people will never forget what you did, but people will never forget how you made them feel." ~ Maya Angelou

Chapter 2

The State of Affairs

Mental illness has become more prevalent over the last few years, encompassing addiction and homelessness. The target population that will be the focus for my clinical experience are those suffering from mental illness and addiction that are admitted to healthcare settings and how we as nurses care for them without sustaining verbal abuse or physical injuries. Healthy People 2020 suggests to "create social and physical environments that promote good health for all", this would include both patients, their families, and nursing staff (Department of Health & Human Services [HHS], 2017, p. 2). In April of this year, the American Nurses Association reported that 62 percent of nurses admitted to being physically injured or physically attacked (American Nurses Association [ANA], 2018, para. 3). Which brings about my focus towards nursing burn out and post-traumatic stress disorder among nurses. The escalation from the patient could be the mental illness, addiction, or even the nurse not being prepared academically from their nursing school or healthcare unit. Because of not being prepared, nurses are unsure how to work with the population and may indirectly cause the escalation that leads to the burn-out and PTSD (Mealer, Burnham, Goode, Rothbaum, & Moss, 2009).

Healthcare's history was primary focused on acute illnesses or injuries (Institute of Medicine [IOM], 2010). As the shift of nursing focuses more on chronic illness, nursing should follow suit with including more mental health care in the nursing curriculum and provide educational programs to help nurses cope with the invisible illness. When researching the National Database of Nursing Quality Indicators (NDNQI), there were a few areas that stood out in regard to the magnitude of the problem. "Registered nurse education, psychiatric physical assault rates, voluntary nursing turnover, and nurse vacancy rate" indicates that these could be related in some way (Montalvo, 2007, figure 1). The question that I would like to base my research on is whether an education plan for nurses will be effective with preventing behavior escalation from patients. The goal is to help patients suffering from mental illness and addiction to receive the care they deserve while giving the nurse tools to create a successful outcome through various coping mechanisms.

The topic of interest and concern is related to the growing problem of violence against nursing staff. When applying workplace violence to the American Association of Colleges of Nursing (AACN) essential number one, one can agree that the underlying foundation applies to the complexity of nursing care (American Association of Colleges of Nursing [AACN], 2006). In preparation for achieving a terminal degree, the AACN introduces concepts that are inline with working with a target population, employing accountability for patient safety by using "communication skills/processes that lead to quality improvement" (AACN, 2006, p. 11). When aligning workplace violence to the essential number one, the focus is on human interaction and identifying safety concerns prior to the behavior escalating (Phillips, 2016). The staff survey data supports the increase of workplace violence and the suggestion of leadership to implement a panel to tackle and formulate a plan to reduce system-wide incidents (Le & Pharm, 2016).

With the evaluation of the literature in comparison to the DNP Essentials, it appears the evidence is recent and applies to the ongoing complexity of workplace violence. Articles received and used for this discussion post reveal the magnitude of workplace violence, mainly in the emergency room and psychiatric units. Violence against nursing staff and nurses is widespread and getting worse. The problem identified for the practicum project is underreporting physical and verbal attacks due to misconceptions of "nothing being done, it is a part of the job, nobody got hurt and appear to look weak among their peers" (Copeland & Henry, 2017, p. 71). Identifying the problem area of hopelessness and burn-out syndrome from the nurses that has led to the theory that workplace violence should be tolerated to some degree has been found that nothing will change if the situation is not reported (Arnetz et al., 2015).

Piecing the Puzzle Together

It is essential to determine the appropriate theory that would encompass the true nature of helping nurses discover ways to work with those who have a mental illness or addiction. The proposed topic took a glance into the current dilemma nurses are facing on healthcare units, and the lack of mental health education nurses receive. Taking this concept and applying the idea of how some nurses behave when stressed out, the patient's behavior could be a direct reflection of how they are acting either by verbal or non-verbal communication. The theory that stands out the most in this situation is Albert Bandura's psychology-based social cognitive theory. The goal is to help nurses to recall situations that they have encountered with escalated behavior while working on a healthcare unit. To create the best practice, it is vital to research all credible information on a topic to create a conclusion that can be utilized. The literature that is obtained "should offer strong support to the current study or project" (Sublett, 2006, p. 63). After all, the research is collected; only the most credible is "synthesized to create recommendations for practice" (Gray, Grove, & Sutherland, 2017, p. 485).

The ending result leads the researcher to have substantial evidence to strengthen the delivery of healthcare. When analyzing the behavior, one thing comes to mind; what was the nurse doing to take control of the situation? The social cognitive theory helps the learner to recognize their behavior, verbal or non-verbal communication, which could bring about a negative response from the escalating patient. By assisting the nurse in controlling their own emotions and behavior can directly result in patient cooperation and higher satisfaction scores (Hodges & Videto, 2011). Methods that the social cognitive theory can be useful in behavior therapy, developing education programs, and learning through observation (Bandura, 2010). Which all three can relate to behavior that we see in the hospital and the creation of an education plan to help nurses understand behavior modification.

Bandura focused on the learner and how they are "actively involved in the environment through personal selection and self-regulation of the learning process through their view of the world" (McEwen & Wills, 2014, p. 399). Applying the theory can help nurses to identify their own emotions or behavior traits, which can help keep the milieu of the unit and help the nurse feel competent in caring for the entire patient. The benefit of keeping the patient calm while in the hospital can help to promote rest and sleep will lead to increased healing and decreased hospitalization (DuBose & Hadi, 2016).

On the flip side, there are times where the patient and their family members are out of control, and the nurse's aid or nurse was not the instigator but the person that absorbed the behavior from these individuals. The behavior could be from finding out a serious medical illness to using medications or illegal substances from the person visiting and bringing them in from outside of the hospital. The nurse has their emotional guard up and nursing license on the line the minute they walk into the doors of the hospital or medical facility that they work. Why is this? Due to the nature of working with mild to severely ill people, there is this level of fearing the unknown. Some are there to malinger, and most patients are not and either suffering somatic complaints or severe injuries or illnesses. By all means, this does not give someone the licenses or permission to treat another person disrespectfully or not. When the nurse is caring for high-stress situations, over a prolonged period, there is no force-field made that can protect the emotional damage that is caused by patients and their families. So modeling the behaviors and having the constant on-edge alertness of the sympathetic nervous system fight or flight response not only eats away at the nurse or healthcare workers' DNA, not only deteriorating their health but for generations to come.

Needs Assessment and Gathering Data

To conduct a needs assessment referencing the cause of patient violence against nurses, would be from several different avenues of gathering information. The first would be through primary data collection of existing research, primarily in the United States, as there is not enough research from each state as of this date. Second, would be from observation of escalation behaviors from the patient and the non-verbal communication the nurse would exhibit during that time. Using observation is key as the nurse may not believe that they could be the contributor to the patient escalating. The third method of gathering info is from one on one interviews of various nurses and group meetings about contributors that could create a hostile work environment for the patient.

Nurses discuss patient challenges with their charge nurses to bounce ideas off the other for the best outcome but also to vent and sometimes release. We have challenging days and assignments where we are expected not to show that we have internalized over the years. These years include no administrative support, made to feel incompetent in our positions, along with the verbal and, at times, physical bashing from patients, their families, and management. It would be irresponsible not to mention that not every administrative body is unsupportive to their staff; some are wonderful and care about the well-being of their employees.

With the on-going stress of the units in mind, it is important to find out as much as we can about a target population, which is nurses, to include nonverbal factors that could contribute to patient behavior escalation (Hodges & Videto, 2011).

The goal is to find the nurse's perceived need and what they feel the need is (Kettner, Moroney, & Martin, 2017). Many nurses have expressed that they are feeling a version of compassion fatigue, which is a "progressive and cumulative process that is influenced by the interactions by patients, the nurse's own resources and exposure to stress" (Mason, Leslie, Lyons, Walke, & Griffin, 2014, p. 217). When considering Maslow's Hierarchy of Needs, various human needs are not being met. The first area would be the physiological needs where nurses work long shifts; some rarely get a drink of water, have a lunch break, or able to use the bathroom.

Second, safety and security, with staying free from injury or unsafe working situations, there are times nurses work short-staffed leaving the nurses overstressed and tired (DeMarco & Tilson, n.d.). Finally, the need to receive respect from the angry patient, family member, and even fellow staff members. There are many aspects of Maslow that correlate well with areas in nursing. Things to consider is the nurse may be missing even the basic needs at work and even at home that could contribute to the unspoken behavior that could cause patient behavior escalation.

Challenges that could occur with obtaining data could involve the nurse feeling as if they are being scrutinized with their practice if they do not understand or open-minded about the reduction of patient on nurse violence. When aiming to achieve a solution, it is necessary to self-reflect with one's practice to ensure all areas are covered that could create a negative outcome when caring for patients. The factor that could also be missing is the nurse may also have undiagnosed or diagnosed mental health conditions that could become aggravated when working under high-stress conditions, mixed with other components of their job.

Chapter 3

The Detriments of Transactional Nursing and Lateral Violence

Patient on nurse violence is growing at an epidemic rate. Recent statistics reflect 62% of nurses have either experienced verbal or physical violence, with approximately 1 in 5 nurses that have been physically assaulted (American Nurses Association [ANA], 2018; Bolvin, 2018). The Joint Commission released a sentinel event eliciting the statistical response from the ANA, which incidents are grossly underreported (The Joint Commission, 2018). Therefore, the real numbers have not yet been identified as nurses fear retaliation. By not having a comprehensive education program for nurses that targets preventing violence in the workplace would help prepare nurses to increase job satisfaction. Other advantages would be to build the nurse-patient relationship with an evidence-based project, and the overall DNP project is on the need for an education program to decrease violent incidences. The goal for this evidence-based project is to find the possible link that incites a negative verbal or physical response from a patient and build a short education program that will benefit both the patient and the nurse during hospitalization. Optimizing the Doctor of Nursing Practice, Essential VI for this project, there is a need to exhibit interprofessional collaboration to improve patient and population outcomes (American Association of Colleges of Nursing [AACN], 2006). By incorporating a psychologist as a preceptor, it has helped find an angle that could help nurses with fine-tuning their communication skills by using a more therapeutic approach. The increased amount of work that nurses are doing on the unit can often create a transactional feeling while caring for our patients. Increased demands must be completed, has decreased the human part of nursing, along with time spent at the bedside. When determining the outcomes for this project, the goal is to increase the therapeutic approach where the patient will become receptive, and it will reduce the amount of anxiety within their visit. Not only will the patient be calmer and receptive to care, but the nurse will also ultimately report a rewarding and satisfying shift.

The application of measurement would include observation of the unit, create a short education in-service on situational anxiety, mental illness, substance abuse, and how or what we say or do can make the shift better. Ultimately by increasing the nurse-patient relationship, it offers the patient security and feelings of having control over their care. To conclude the evaluation of the education piece, observation, and a simple survey would be given for feedback. The details would include how the nurse feels about their shift and how the education for this project helped them. By offering this education piece, it may enhance and improve the organizational culture, by altering the shared behaviors on the unit about caring for someone that may seem difficult (White, Dudley-Brown, & Terhaar, 2016). A healthcare provider that can "explain, listen, and empathize significantly affects the biological and functional outcomes and influences a patient's perception of care and satisfaction measures" (Institute for Healthcare Communication, 2011, p. 358). As a result, we could anticipate the nurse to report an uneventful, satisfied, and a seemingly rewarding shift by increasing the human and decreasing the feeling of a transactional approach.

To state that the patient and nurse relationship is vital in the delivery of care is also the one that must abide by their position on the subject matter. I love difficult patients and helping nurses understand by taking this bear of a patient on for my assignment is that it is not always the patient that has the behavior. The point is that we are swamped, have many tasks to perform for five to seven patients at a time, where did we start losing the human side to our care? Could being goal-driven and focused be a detriment to the nurse-patient relationship? Over time this non-stop high-energy nursing begins to wear down on nurses to where they innocently forget the people side to patient care, otherwise known as compassion fatigue, burn-out and post-traumatic stress disorder (PTSD) (Mealer, Burnham, Goode, Rothbaum, & Moss, 2009; Mason, Leslie, Lyons, Walke, & Griffin, 2014). Our shift tasks are essential, but so is having a relationship with the patient to not only fulfill your duties as a nurse, without injury but to enjoy and love your job. Just to change things up a little, one week in clinical I decided to perform a mini-experiment along with the therapeutic communication techniques. The goal was to introduce smiling more into the equation by actively listening to the patient. Most communication methods in a stressful environment in the workplace can appear more transactional, and the perception from the patient is the nurse is not paying attention or listening to their concerns (Wienclaw, 2017). Nonverbal and verbal communication can translate into a misunderstanding when a patient is not feeling well. By changing how we perceive ourselves in this process, can significantly affect our relationship with the patient as what we say or do may be misinterpreted. Gathering this information was crucial to this project.

One of the best solutions to this epidemic has brought many researchers, healthcare authorities and authors to conclude that a prevention plan should be implemented to prevent issues. Researching various programs out on the market, including government initiatives, prevention has not been the focus and identified as psychiatric physical violence as being a problem. Mental health experts argue that de-escalation is the key to every situation and is the prevention plan. According to the Oxford journal, de-escalation begins when the patient or their family member has already started cursing and showing pronounce agitation versus prevention is not allowing the behavior to get to this point. What is really the problem? The evidence is pointing at unruly behavior from patients, their families, and between staff members, but why? There are many pieces to this puzzle, and many points to the direction of lack of building professional boundaries, relationships, and trust between the healthcare system, those we serve, and between workers. This is a systematic hole and failure.

"Whether you think you can, or you think you can't…You're Right!" ~Henry Ford

Chapter 4

Electronic Medical Records and the Insufficiency Pathway

The use of a health information system (HIS) can be beneficial for an organization, yet also severe if it is not maintained or thoughtful consideration put into the design for the organization. Limitations of not having or having a minimal computerized health information system can include organization difficulties, increased medical errors, poor data tracking, and an increase in human error (Yusof & Sahroni, 2018). Without the ability to track the progress of a project with the accuracy of obtaining electronic data, it hinders the phases of project management (White, Dudley-Brown, & Terhaar, 2016). A quality health information system needs to be updated frequently to keep up with the changes in healthcare, including the varying patient acuity. Future planning of projects could be impacted as data would be managed through Excel spreadsheets and graphs, which could be simplified if data was captured and integrated regularly.

When referring to the implementation of the EMR, it was designed to decrease near-misses and to gather data. The integration of a health information system requires appropriate training of the system. However, if there is no data or even incidents occurring on the floor, nothing is being captured. When the incident happens, and the information is not entered into the system, the person gathering the reports for management review, the EMR system, more times than not, it will not reveal workplace violence situations, as no report was or designated folder for these events. If it is not reported or discovered, the incident never happened. The benefit of having a HIS is increased organization within the health care system, greater efficiency of patient care, and data capture to view if new interventions or processes are gearing towards effective change. As a bonus, the "pay for performance (P4P)" can assist in the implementation of new and updating systems to "improve healthcare efficiency and quality" (Kondo et al., 2016, p. S61).

The implications for not implementing a computerized charting system in a larger setting can range from errors to fraud and abuse of the healthcare system, resulting in higher costs for consumers (Bowman, 2013). The use of a Health Information Exchange (HIE) organization could be a benefit or not when it comes to patient perception. Purpose of the HIE organization sends patient information across the country to various local and state organizations to trading partners, other care providers, laboratories, inpatient facilities, and not limited giving information to just patients (The Office of the National Coordinator for Health Information Technology, 2017). When taking this a step farther, is it unethical for businesses to not give access to employees to report violent incidents from patients, their families, or from staff, including upper management? Absolutely! It has been a requirement from both the Joint Commission and Occupational Safety and Health Administration (OSHA) for facilities to report incidents and without retaliation, with the whistleblower hotline service that OSHA provides. What I recently discovered, the OSHA central Florida office that is located in the Tampa area, the department that handles retaliation, is closed due to funding. Taking another step to see the available resources, the Equal Opportunity Employee Commission (EEOC) stated that they could only work with cases relating to discrimination.

Barriers of Reporting Workplace Violence

The barrier to reporting is far more complicated than initially thought, as the current research is unveiling a twist. When digging into the nurse's belief system about reporting incidents, the statements have been collected that being injured is a part of the job and that reporting anything does not make a difference (Copeland & Henry, 2017).

Under the workplace violence protocol, which is system-wide, it makes the statement of notifying the nurse manager or if they are not available to contact the administrator on duty. The computerized reporting system does not state anything that references the report of a workplace violence incident and is primarily under the "miscellaneous" tab. If a nurse reports the kick, slap, or punch, they can note it in the system. The reporting system then sends an email report to the administration, the nurse manager, and risk management. Incidents are discussed in a meeting that focuses on specific issues that the director of nursing finds to be an issue. There was an opportunity for me to listen to a meeting outlining the problems or concerns from the nurse managers to the administration team about current affairs and statistics. While sitting there, observing the structure of the meeting, there was a massive disconnect between the admin team versus the floor managers. They did not want to hear anything except medication variances, falls, and pressure ulcer statistics. Nothing was brought up about violence on the floors. They even homed in on a near miss but never asked about how the admin team could help the situation, only delegated more transactions and surveying of the problem.

The leg that I was working on for the first section of my project was about reporting measures and why nurses and nursing staff were not reporting incidents. It was a goal of mine, just to see if I was imagining the violence happening on the units. The idea consisted of a balloting system where the staff could do an anonymous survey and fill out a short 30-second paper after each incident, that is kept anonymous, stating the kind of injury, what shift, how it happened, and if they felt safe. The first week, one person filled it out. The second week it was a 900% increase, mostly consisting of verbal incidents and one person that had multiple events, as mentioned by the nurse manager that was assisting me with this data collection. During this time, these areas that I was working on were for my DNP project, which was opening and closing doors simultaneously. I was chosen to serve on the End Nurse Abuse campaign with the American Nurses Association (ANA), this was not only a huge honor but something that I felt was where I took ownership and felt that I could make the difference. Coincidentally, the Joint Commission came out with sentinel event #59 "Physical and verbal violence against healthcare workers," where the ANA responded with the End Nurse Abuse Advisory Committee! As outlined in the statement by the Joint Commission, they stated that issues were not only required to be reported, but incidents were vastly underreported due to nurses feeling retaliated against or made to believe that violence is a part of the job.

    I rushed to call my preceptor as fast as I could, she was excited, and we talked about expanding the anonymous reporting ballot box. The next day or two, she came and told me that four other departments were on board. The day before we were going to implement these changes, I received a phone call that changed everything, I was excused from my rotation. The intention was not to penalize anyone or institution but to help internally and possibly create a position for myself to help make things better. Nothing more, nothing less. What it did do was make my life hell as I was laughed at, told that it was a great topic, but "diving in a pool of black tar," everything that would make most people cringe, only reinforced why I had to stand firm. Looking into the research obtained, there was so much literature discussing the same slogans over and over again, "Violence is a part of the job," "Nothing will ever get done," this had to be something to focus on, a change needed to happen.

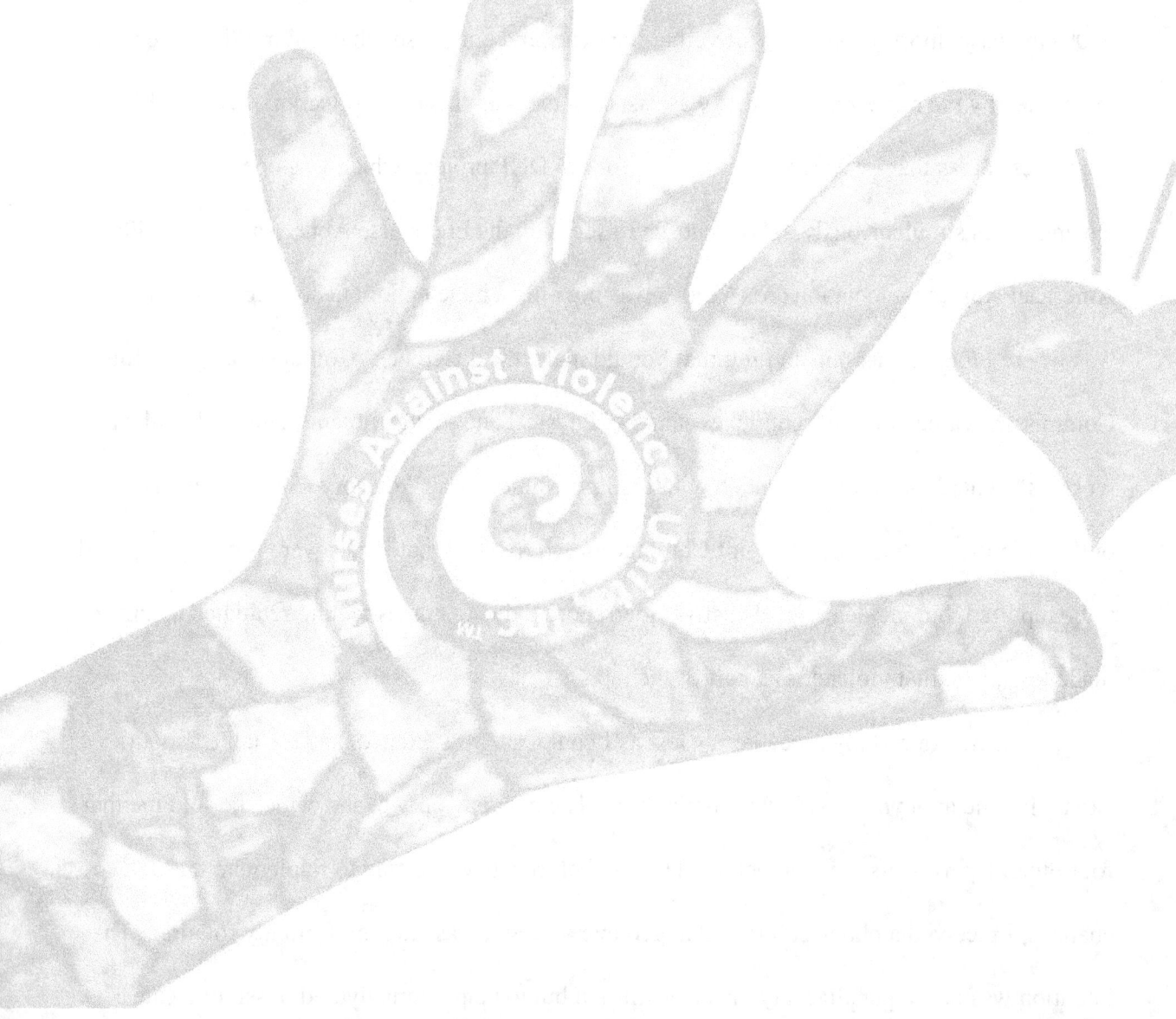

Chapter 5

The Discovery

One could believe that the floors do not have any issues with the patient on nurse violence, or they could dig a little deeper to find out why. When investigating the process of reporting, it was discovered that if a nurse or staff member reported an incident to the charge nurse, nurse manager, or the administrator on duty during the nighttime, the event was not recorded unless it was a code. During shift report, the nurse passed it in report about the patient being combative, then charge nurse is aware but no safeguards are in place to protect that nurse. It is not the nurse leaving that is held responsible for passing the patient off to the oncoming shift. The off-going nurse believes that they are doing the right thing by notifying all those in charge and filing a report. What was discovered during this rotation is that when the report is entered in the online reporting system or verbally told the nurse manager or the administrator on duty, they are not keeping tallies for data collection of incidents that are happening on the floor.

Observed Activity

Through many years of personal and statements from fellow nurses over the years, patient on nurse violence has grown to epidemic proportions. The research that was done independently did not measure the magnitude of the problem. When talking with the nurses on the floor and charge nurse, the story was standard, that the staff nurse would report a violent patient to the charge nurse, nurse manager, or the administrator on duty (AOD) at night. Unless a violent patient code was called, a report would not be done by the AOD, the only person that writes the report. The computer reporting system did not have a link to report workplace violence so that the nurse would report it as a miscellaneous problem. The computerized report would be sent to the top administration, and the nurse manager to work on a resolution to the problem at the "First Focus" meeting that is held once a week. When I had the opportunity to go, there were only a select few issues that were covered, and the nurse manager had to offer the resolution to the issue. When I asked my preceptor if she could pull data for behavior escalation issues resulting in verbal or physical assault, there was no data to be found. Which had resulted in creating a ballot system for nurses to fill out little slips whenever there was an incident, along with a survey about their mental health education in nursing school, and various issues that have happened caused by patients.

All the surveys requested a forum to discuss the patients that they are working with and how to manage them without becoming burned out from the behavior. In the staff meeting, the system was introduced. The nurses were receptive for the most part and accepted the system to see how much is going on. In two days, there was a 100% increase in reporting a verbal incident. The next week a 900% increase, involving five incidents, nine verbal and 6 of those, physically assaulted a nurse. Out of the ten assaults, three did not feel safe working with the individual or for their personal safety off the clock. The fourth week, reporting slouched and slips were not filled out. The nurses were re-educated and encouraged to report to gather data. To do a buddy system if need be, where if one nurse is slammed, the charge nurse could write out the slip.

Evidence-Based Practice

As previously mentioned, if the problem is not reported, there will be no data. Therefore, nothing happened. The lack of reporting reinforces to the violent patient that the behavior is acceptable, and the behavior will continue (Arnetz et al., 2015). The nurse adapts to the bad behavior and the belief of being hurt on the job, cursed at, or feeling inadequate to care for the patient exhibiting behavior issues, is a normal part of the job (Chapman, Styles, Perry, & Combs, 2010). The nurses that are on the unit show a large amount of resilience with facilitating our roles and desire to increase a positive "outcome of wellness" for these individuals (Polk, 1997, p. 2).

The main theory that stands out with my personal experience is how to work with those that have been incarcerated, using the criminology theory. To work with those that are acutely mentally ill is to be open to the fact that they may have a criminal background and are unable to adjust to a stable way of life. The one thing that stands out the most with every acute mental health episode or events leading up to it starts with the patient trying to manipulate the nurse for more medications, mainly opioids. Most of the time the patient is not on any mental health medications and homeless, so the incidence of an outburst is high. The criminology theory points out that nurses and police officers have the same type of patients, just the police have more experience with working with the behaviors to receive cooperation (Henson, 2010). The last part of the practicum project will be an informational forum to discuss the findings, discuss the concepts of a modified therapeutic communication, and a schematic for the charge nurses to use for staffing.

New Literature and Evidence

The latest research found about reporting incidents were a few from an American hospital system, and the other was another country, only two proved to be the most relevant, ironically from the same authors from Detroit. When conducting recent research, it was through a combined search engine CINAHL and Medline for reporting workplace violence. The first article discusses how there is a "lack of systemic, systematic surveillance of violent incidents, including the lack of basic data that could inform administrators" about the safety concerns that nurses and nursing staff are facing (Arnetz et al., 2013, p. 52). The second article remarks about underreporting the patient on nurse workplace violence, that "it creates an underestimation of the true extent of the problem" (Arnetz et al., 2015, p. 200). Furthermore, without accurate data, the problem cannot be addressed to the capacity as it should as the information is incongruent to what is happening in all medical units.

To find the holes and gaps of reporting, my preceptor allowed me to create a workplace violence box where the nurses could fill out a slip of paper of the issue and put it in anonymously, so they would not feel pressured or obligated. The monthly staff meeting was the unveiling; the nurses were very interested. A brief introduction to the project was given, and questions were answered. The study was followed up by an email from the preceptor to all staff to help obtain numbers for data. A few days went by, and the next clinical day we had a 100% increase in data, which was only one, a verbal assault from a 38-year-old male. In addition to the voluntary slips for reporting incidents, I also implemented a survey to find out the background of those participating in the study. There were five respondents in a week, all nurses giving their frank opinions from prompted questions about the current reporting system, how much mental health training in school and the workplace, how often they are attacked or verbally assaulted, and if they would be receptive to an educational forum. The statistics are overwhelming with wanting an educational forum, and the history of verbal and physical assaults go back countless years with worries about their safety moving forward.

When applying the principles of evidence-based practice to violence against nurses, it is important first to analyze the type of patient, the nurses time, patient load, organizational support system, and the amount of knowledge to care for those that have an underlying mental health condition or addiction issue. Most nurses have reported during the research window that they had a range of two weeks to two months, varying on the year they went to nursing school and the curriculum benchmarks from the board of nursing. Without knowledge other than the basic therapeutic communication, nurses have either forgotten how to communicate or get nervous when a patient is verbally or physically aggressive. There has been a study that verbal or other violence on hospital units "decreased by 45% following education" (Adams, Roddy, Knowles, Ashworth, & Irons, n.d., p. 12). Preventing the problem, incorporating education, and reporting the verbal and physical abuse, will eventually reduce nurse stress and increase productivity (Gates, Gillespie, & Succop, 2011).

Exploring the Change Theory aka Criminology Theory

With the increase of violence in the workplace from both personal experience and those involved in the current practicum study. The study correlates the similarities with what police experience to what the nursing profession experiences in the hospital and other areas of healthcare. When looking at the base of this theory, it discusses the "lack of crime prevention and expertise which impedes on the nurse to fully incorporate in prevention techniques" (Henson, 2010, p. 555-556). After having personal experience with incarcerated individuals, this has been the ongoing theme in subsequent years that patients are often behaving like criminals when they act out and become violent with staff. The current workplace policy states that there will be a de-escalation class offered if the individual chooses to take it. The goal is to prevent the problems before escalation, to keep a calm unit, and ensure a safe environment for the patient, nurse, and nursing staff.

Summation

When the reporting gap was discovered, it was apparent that to have a successful practicum rotation that one would need to tread carefully as this is a significant finding in a large hospital system. The goals for the second application is to obtain data of the verbal and physical abuse, observe the interactions, and formulate a teaching plan to provide the nurses on the unit in a forum. As nerve wrecking and upsetting to find this gap, it is important and will not only save a good nurse from burnout, but also increase safety for all, and assist the corporation in their bottom line financially.

The goal of the evidence-based practice practicum project is to focus on the prevalence of patient to nurse violence in the workplace. The beginning steps would include identifying the number of behavior issues that the facility reports through their internal data sources. When conducting independent research about the patient on nurse violence, the numbers are staggering as every report reflects the statistics differently. One article stated that "13 percent of nurses report physical abuse each year", this number appears to be incongruent to the "80 percent of emergency room nurses that experience physical violence during their careers" (Advisory Board, 2016). Most of the statistical data about violence against nurses were minimal, outdated or only reflecting the emergency room data. Literature evidence suggests reporting verbal abuse and violent acts, whereas, on the medical units, nurses that are giving direct patient care are not reporting incidents.

Contributing factors to under-reporting incidents can be related to the misconception that either nothing will be done or that it is a part of the job. Furthermore, nurses have stated that they are fearful of retaliation from their employer, black-listed for having an injury or unable to obtain a new job due to reporting the injury and looking weak among peers (Copeland & Henry, 2017).

Mental health and addiction challenges are prevalent in every healthcare unit and specialty. A good number of individuals suffer from some form of situational anxiety when admitted to the hospital admission or by visiting a family member (Gullich, Ramos, Anschau Zan, Scherer, & Mendoza-Sassi, 2013). The reporting of incidents is essential to obtain information on workplace violence but to also keep a safe environment for both staff and patients. Bottom line, if there is some form of battery that results in or comes close to an injury or verbal assault if it is not reported, it is regarded as it did not happen (Arnetz et al., 2015). One of the most significant challenges will be to break through the nurse's belief system, provide an educational focus group. By having this resource available to staff, it will allow everyone to include information and express concerns about the current system. The benefit to the nurse participating is the recognition of their behaviors regarding reporting, and that is the only barrier, the fear of retaliation (Chen, Huang, Hwang, & Chen, 2010). All in all, if the administration does not have the data, then there will be no evidence of a problem. Ultimately leading to more of the same, inadequate coverage, which results in nurse burn-out and injuries from patients.

Workplace violence is on the rise and an end is nowhere in sight. The main component of the epidemic is the lack of effective communication which exemplifies the problem of reporting the patient on nurse abuse. Being an active, and engaged leader, it is vital to bring forth effective communication that will result in the reduction of burnout and increase errors in the workplace (White, Dudley-Brown, & Terhaar, 2016). The focus of reducing injuries and escalation from the person that is addicted to substances, alcohol, or have an underlying mental health disorder, is to "provide care that is responsive to patient preferences, needs and values" (Grindel, 2016, p. 11). The care that they are receiving may not be the care that they desire for their addiction but focused around the medical issue and why they are admitted. Communication with someone that has a history of escalation, demands, addiction, and mental health conditions is different. The patient attempts several methods of manipulation, while reading the nurse's behavior for weak points of communication. As nurses, we care, bottom line, but are we inconsistent with the care that we give. It is hard to keep continuity of care with the ever-changing patient assignments and for those that have never worked with inmates or mental health patients, it can be difficult.

Chapter 6

Theoretical Basis

The goal is to increase the communication to be not only effective, but to prevent and reduce the number of incidents on the hospital units. It can be achieved by allowing the patient voice their concerns about the situation that are experiencing, as it allows them to feel more in control. When the nurse communicates with the patient, it is vital to be empathetic, kind, and consistent by doing the same thing every time with every patient (Kennealy, Skeem, Manchak, & Louden, 2012). As nurses, we have learned how to use therapeutic communication during in nursing school, and it is rarely remembered during a crisis event. The other issue is that nurses are overloaded and do not recognize the cues due to the demands from their work assignment. As a result, the situation becomes escalated and the other patients on the nurse's assignment are not receiving the care that they need. The goal for using the criminology theory, is to emphasize the importance of setting rules for conduct, and consequences if the rules are broken (Henson, 2010). When combined with adaptation, the nurse can "maintain their emotional well-being and psychological self by employing self-protection" (Chapman, Styles, Perry, & Combs, 2010, p. 186). When laying the foundation of remaining empathetic, yet firm, fair, and consistent, the patient with high-level needs will be unable to split staff, manipulate, or lead to nursing burnout, which is achieved by not letting the patient break the environment of unity.

During onsite clinicals, it is evident that nurses and nursing staff through both indirect and direct communication via surveys or personal interviews; are looking for ways to decrease the patient on nurse violence on their unit. The ballot system is a new reporting method that has taken some time to truly breakthrough previous beliefs about reporting verbal and physical violence on the units. The reasoning is due to the hole in communication, where the nurse would report it and it would end in a verbal report, without documentation. Without data, there are no problems to report. Breaking through the ongoing statements of nothing being done, nurses are right in many ways. Especially if the data is not there to support the claims. To ensure that information is being transferred and reported, this will be the toughest challenge to overcome.

Social Cognitive Theory

It is apparent that nurses have learned through "direct experiences, human dialog, and interaction" through various situations and with abusive patients (White, Dudley-Brown, & Terhaar, 2016, p. 62). The social cognitive theory is most appropriate and especially helpful with the upcoming creation of the educational piece to the DNP project, as it focuses on behavior modification and introducing new information into practice. For example, the power of monitoring ones' own behavior can reveal the environment and cognitive conditions from the nurse, which could result in poor morale on the unit and negative behavior toward reporting incidents (Bandura, 2001). In so many words, nurses can create their own environment through influencing the outcome (Lasater, Mood, Buchwach, & Dieckmann, 2015).

The goal is to break through the previous thoughts patterns about reporting verbal and physical assaults and provide an easy reporting method that would result in data collection without feelings of workplace retaliation. Encouraging the nurse to report workplace violence will enable them to not only feel empowered but create the culture of safety through an easier reporting system, without the result of punitive administrative action. The anonymous balloting system appears to be simple and allowing the busy nurse to complete it without filling out long reports which are not connected to a data collection unit. The social cognitive theory will assist the nurse with the plan of overcoming their personal feelings and address the rising violence from patients. Once this goal is achieved, the nurse learners will build more confidence in the reporting system and see a more positive unit as a result of acuity-based staffing. The criminology theory is valid, but it will be the and adaptation and social cognitive theory that will be the catalyst for the education piece of my DNP project.

Evaluation of Outcomes

- Creates the culture of reporting patient on nurse aggression.
- Acuity to staffing protocols shift to accommodate the patient load.
- Nursing burn-out, turn-over, & nursing injuries decrease.
- Patient satisfaction scores go up.
- Job satisfaction scores go up, resulting in nurse retention.

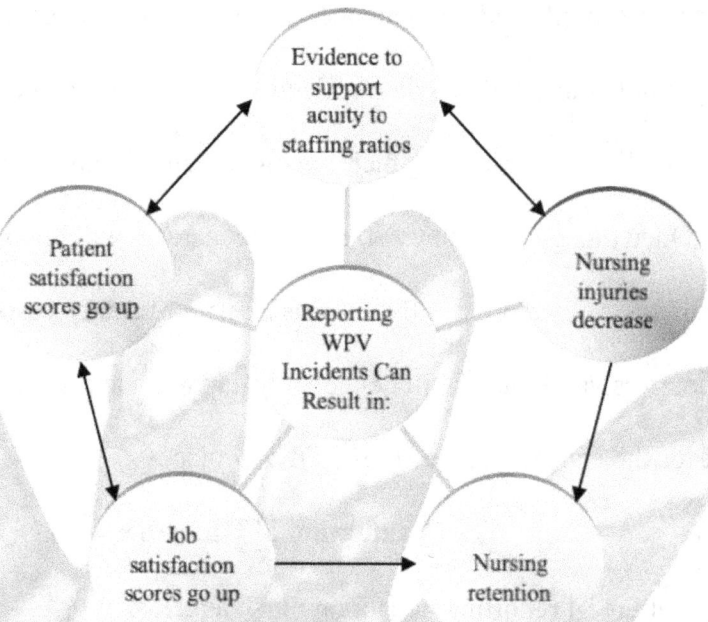

The method of evaluating the outcomes begins when the nurse reports the workplace violence incident. When the anonymous data is collected about the incident by using a ballot box, the nurse fills in the shift, type of assault, age, date of the incident, and if the member feels safe. The ballots are then collected, tallied using a spreadsheet method, separated by the week, age of patient, violent episode, and shift. Without collecting data, a violence prevention program, preventions, or protections for the nursing staff cannot be "customized and target the high-risk areas" (McPhaul, London, & Lipscomb, 2013, p. 4). Evaluating the outcome of reporting will also involve nursing staff participation in reporting incidents, contributing to the goal of nurse retention. Measurement of the psychosocial outcome can be achieved through evaluating the "moods, attitudes, and ability to interact with others" (White, Dudley-Brown, & Terhaar, 2016, p. 76).

Proposal of new guidelines:

Practice guidelines would include various areas of improvement. The first would include the mandatory reporting of all workplace violence incidents, with a non-purgatory and short reporting system. Propose a mental health professional to float on the units to sit and talk with the potential violent or those that are exhibiting increased stress and anxiety symptoms. Introduce an educational plan and forum that can help the nurses and nursing staff to communicate effectively with all patients, including those with mental illness. Finally, to help create the culture of personal safety and mental health by introducing the concept of time-outs for those affected by unit violence.

Standards of care:

The standards of care should mimic those of the proposed practice guidelines, as there is a wide-open hole of lacking data that contributes to the circle of events. The national standard for employers should be the enforcement of the zero-tolerance policy that does not involve punitive retaliation to the reporting nurse, whether injured or not (The Joint Commission, 2018). Cutting through the behavior adaptation from the nurses with the physical and verbal abuse, a system needs to be in place that focuses on rebuilding nursing confidence, and creating a culture of reporting (Chapman, Styles, Perry, & Combs, 2010). The nursing staff will not only begin to appreciate the new measures, it will show through their performance, and affect in the unit. As a result, the patient satisfaction scores will go up, and the departments will retain their nurses.

Outcome:

The key of prevention is knowledge. Utilizing the practice strategies with a modified form of therapeutic communication, the efforts will bring about positive change and reduction of violent outbursts from the patient, resulting in higher patient satisfaction scores. The new practice strategies will be achieved when nurses understand the simple concepts that can reduce aggression on the units. As a result, the hospital system will see an increase of job satisfaction, staff retention, lower the overall expenditures related to near misses, misses due to fatigue, and workplace violence.

Proposed practice approach:

A modified therapeutic communication by utilizing empathy with the firm, fair, and consistent method. Working closely with patients and nurses for over a quarter of a century, the one thing that has been amplified over the years is the desire to always do good for the patient. When a patient is angry, the nurse often takes it to heart or tries to make the patient feel better, this is what we do. In combination with reporting the verbal and physical escalation, the goal is to implement a modified therapeutic communication method that will help diffuse the situation before it happens.

"The more you care, the stronger you can be." ~Jim Rohn

Chapter 7

Advocating Policy Changes

If the policy is not broken, add to it. If the policy is promoting either direct or indirect harm, it would be detrimental to those that it affects to keep it. Standardization is key when implementing an "ethically sound framework that focuses on quality measures" and the safety of both patients and nursing staff (Suchy, 2010, p. 242). When working with a critical area that is underreported, such as the patient on nurse violence, it is difficult for policymakers in the organization to know what is going on if incidents are not being reported (Arnetz et al., 2015). One of the benefits of working on WPV in nursing in the practicum setting is close access to the problem area and able to build relationships with the nursing staff. A huge problem over the years has been the feeling that administration is not doing anything about the escalating violence, so what is the point of even trying to report anything. Being a nursing leader and working closely with the staff is providing them with an ear to talk about their experiences without feeling penalized or inadequate as a nurse.

The implementation of new evidence-based practices should be reviewed by policymakers as old policies may not always fit the ever-changing healthcare systems. For example, there is a great concern about the lack of quality through inefficiency, systematic evaluation, and insufficient staffing (Izumi, 2013). If the policies remain the same, the three areas would not only worsen but place not only the patient at risk but also those that are caring for them. While searching for my practicum setting policies on workplace violence, there was only one standardized policy across the system. All the others relating to violent patients were only in certain hospitals and not system wide. The WPV policy did not list a solution except for the nurse that suffered the incident to report the issue to the charge nurse, nurse manager, or administrator on duty. If the nurse did not fill out a computerized report, then the only one that knows is the next shift, that may or may not keep reporting the problem. Finding the evidence of a problem is key, then tracing the steps through the process to see if there can be any improvements made and report the findings after extensive research to make your case to the board of directors. To be a leader in nursing, it takes time, consistency, and a passion for doing what is right.

Policy Development

To implement a policy, developing research priorities must be on the forefront to discover the institutional problem (Rehfuess et al., 2016). In health care facilities in general, it is known that patients are hurting nurses either directly or indirectly through escalated events. To effectively get through to policy makers, the researcher needs to be aware of current policies, how the system operates, the economic factors (Harrington, Crider, Benner, & Malone, 2005). The first step of collecting data is by using a survey on the unit; this can point out the issues stand out in practice. Next, to see how much escalation is currently happening through a balloting system, as data reflecting workplace violence is virtually nonexistent. Last, develop a plan to reveal data to the policy makers with an education plan that discusses the modified therapeutic communication method, and increase the access to an easier reporting system so the numbers will be accurate. The goal is to translate the evidence gathered from the study into an organized framework, such as blending the criminology and adaptation theory into a personal safety theory (White, Dudley-Brown, & Terhaar, 2016). Becoming a leader in nursing and the community requires one to push forward through tough circumstances to not only grow but positively affect those around them. Nursing has a vast array of knowledge to be learned, applied, and revisited to incorporate new concepts and ideas into practice. As a nursing leader, it is a nursing privilege and personal obligation to find weaker areas that affect the safety of the patient and nursing staff by implementing initiatives into practice (Grindel, 2016). The most recent economic statistics regarding workplace violence cites an "estimated $121 billion a year" across the nation, and "more than 876,000 lost workdays, with $16 million lost wages" (Nixon, 2018, para. 7). The numbers would include the patient violence against nurses if the assaults were reported. That number would be much higher from current data estimation from the practicum rotation.

Future plans that encompass healthcare advocacy and helping to develop policy, is to continue to hold firm with the teaching program that branched out from this project. The goal is to continue helping nurses to receive education about mental illness and addiction, in hopes to help nurses remain safe, and free from mental and physical abuse. I am working with a psychologist to strengthen my position in effort to mesh psychology and nursing together and help nurses from education to a free to low cost therapy service. I believe that the DNP program has helped me to strengthen ideas and give me the confidence that I need to be recognized as a leader within the nursing field. The difference between this term and the past clinical experiences from about a year ago, is that I was not as prepared or solid in a position to discuss ideas with my preceptor freely and without feeling persecuted. Patient on violence is a topic that does not sit well with administration, at least at the one healthcare facility where I was excused from. It was a tough road, but I am here. As a result of being blacklisted from the hospital system, I moved towards Orlando to find a DNP to work with and the help of the other preceptor, a psychologist in Tampa. Life is certainly busy these days but feel blessed that I have the best of both worlds to help me with the DNP journey.

Strategies to Overcome Barriers

Barriers can be an issue with a hot topic such as patient violence on nurses and other staff members. The costs associated with replacing nurses due to injury, worker's compensation, and nursing turnover are massive. To replace a nurse, OSHA reports that is costs an estimated "$27,000 to 103,000 which includes separation, recruiting, hiring, orientation, and training" (Occupational Safety and Health Administration [OSHA], n.d., p. 4). If the hospital replaced 20 nurses, it would cost them approximately 2,060,000 according to the data provided. The cost does not include time lost, injuries, and worker's compensation costs. The cost per day that the non-profit hospital receives for basic care from insurance companies, in Florida, was approximately $2,224 per patient (Rappleye, 2015, p. 2). When you factor $2,224 x 365 days, that totals $811,760 if a patient was admitted all year. The average hospital census is approximately 80 patients, so the hospital makes with basic care alone is $177,920 per day, averaging about $64,940,800 per year, for a basic hospital stay.

The first barrier that can be overcome is pointing out the costs for injuries of staff, time off, worker's compensation claims, and nursing turnover rates in comparison to the amount of money that is pulled in from basic patient care. The next barrier to overcome is to show evidence of the length of the computerized reporting system, and the current hole in the system that the data is not being recorded. Exemplifying the benefits of implementing a teaching plan with modified therapeutic communication techniques that will help nurses work with mental health and addiction patients, and the ease of reporting data. The data captured will show the magnitude of the issue and then a gradual decrease to elimination of abuse on the units, and not just in the emergency department. The goal is to convey the importance of reporting and to have an open dialog with nurses that creates a conducive environment of personal safety while caring for those that suffer from addictions or mental illness, through awareness and knowledge. Through using these techniques and suggestions, it will help the nurse feel supported and job satisfaction will increase. The main teaching component will be developed for this DNP project.

Practicum Professional Development Objectives

By the end of this practicum, the DNP level nurse will be able to:

1. Analyze and dissect the current information about the ease of reporting procedures.
2. Evaluate the learner's understanding about reporting procedures.
3. Create an educational forum to improve understanding about reporting procedures with an increase in workplace violence reporting.

Learning Objectives

By the end of the project, the DNP level student will be able to:

1. Facilitate the learner by helping them interpret the learned material to work and life experiences with those that have mental health challenges.
2. Facilitate the learner to compare patient scenarios, dissect information to fit the situation, and aim to keep the milieu of the unit.

3. Generate a simple plan that will increase unit morale, by bringing awareness to the increase of workplace violence through reporting the incidents.

4. Analyze and dissect the current information about the ease of reporting procedures.

Knowledge is the root of theory in combination with various additional research, which backs up evidence-based practice when used in the clinical setting. Bringing in previously learned material from a wide variety of current or past experiences, contributes to finding a solution or add knowledge to a certain situation (Fawcett & Garity, 2009). When applying all learned knowledge to an area, the ideas and statements defines the concept, or theory that are concrete in and specific in nature (Fawcett & Garity, 2009). Nursing research takes the knowledge and theory that is specific to a certain area in nursing, conducts a systematic search focusing on "analyzing phenomenon" and applies the information to improve the practice (Fawcett & Garity, 2009, p. 5). When the research is complete, and all areas are explored, evidence-based practice will "integrate the best research with a combination of clinical expertise, to deliver quality, and cost-effective care to the patient" (Gray, Grove, & Sutherland, 2017, p. 18).

The relationship between knowledge, theory, research and evidence-based practice is the use of the best practices and quality outcomes for the patient. Using knowledge of the violence that nurses face on the units with firsthand, helps to determine the right method of approach, or theory that is needed to gain support from the nurses for this evidenced-based project. Research of the current policies in place, along with the reporting system, will enhance the theory and support the knowledge previously learned. The current system is a failure as the protocol for both reporting and workplace violence, do not provide data, as there is not a place to report patients attacking staff. The quality measurement that is currently in use is notifying the administrator on duty, and if there is a code, then a report is filled out. Without a reporting system for quality control purposes, the problem does not exist. The use of quality improvement measurements can assist in the evaluation of the problem area, then devise a plan to implement evidence-based practices that will result in a reduction of nurses being attacked or injured (Djulbegovic, 2014).

"How very little can be done under the spirit of fear." ~ Florence Nightingale

Chapter 8

Evidence-Based Model

When determining the evidence-based model in the practicum setting, it is important to look at the whole picture of a situation prior to development. The Iowa model appears to stand out the most in this practicum setting but still has major deficits when used with patient to nurse violence. The focus of this practicum project is underreported incidents, barriers preventing reporting, and the lack of data showing the violence on the floors. The goal is to break through the stigma of reporting a slap, kick, spit, or scratching episode and verbally threatening behavior; and help the nurses understand that not reporting the problem will not provide data for correction. The "Iowa model focuses on collaboration in the use of research" which also helps to "identify triggers" of areas that need improvement (Doody & Doody, 2011, p. 661). It is reasonable to assume that the model to continue the research for reporting patient on nurse violence will continue with using the Iowa model by monitoring the progress of reporting patient on nurse violence, monitor changes in practice, and filter out the results of progress (Gray, Grove, & Sutherland, 2017, p. 483).

Adoption of New Approaches

The use of conceptual maps is amazing as they "summarize and integrate" new information to help the learner to understand new concepts of a study (Gray et al., 2017, p. 140). During the last clinical day, a discovery was made that the computerized reporting system was not user-friendly and there was no data collection persay about workplace violence. The common theme across nursing is if you report it, nothing will get done or that the physical and verbal abuse that they are receiving is a part of the job (Phillips, 2016). When clinical and floor experience collide with the statements of nothing being done if something is being reported, it was a huge curiosity that involved reviewing the process of the regular reporting system (Rosswurm & Larrabee, 1999). The system did not have a column for workplace violence to separate and signal that there is a problem. When the floor nurse has a problem with a patient attack, the nurse manager or administrator on duty is notified and if there is a code, the paperwork is filled out and a report is made. If a nurse reports it on the reporting system, the nurse manager and others see it but there is no data obtained or tracking of verbal or physical assaults. They float away after being addressed, if reported. The common statement of nothing will get done if someone reports something does have a validity. All in all, the biggest challenge is to create a system that takes a little time for the floor nurse and to help them feel that they will not be retaliated against.

Reflection of Professional Experience

Workplace violence is trending upwards in recent years than in previous years. The latest statistics noted that "39% of nurses reported verbal assaults whereas, only 13% report physical abuse each year" (Advisory Board, 2016, para. 3). Throughout my nursing career, there have been multiple times where nurses have been yelled at and hurt. The common theme about nursing is that it is a tough job that requires thick skin that can handle verbal berating and threats. When asking nurses if they have been hurt or threatened by a competent patient and they will boldly tell you that it is a part of the job, "would be received as weak by peers, nobody was hurt," and why bother reporting it because nothing ever gets done (Copeland & Henry, 2017, p. 71). Breaking through the misconceptions is one of the main goals for this practicum project.

Observation

During the observation of the medical unit, it is noticeable that it is very busy, the staff is attentive to call bells, and the nurse manager even helps to toilet people throughout her day. The teamwork is noticeable. The nurse manager has stated that there has been an overwhelming amount of outburst and behavior issues from patients over the last few months that has even led to a nurse filing stalking charges against a patient's family member. One of the staff nurses had an issue where the patient that was diagnosed with dementia, attempted to punch her while trying to assist him to the bathroom. The nurse stated that the "patient punched me, but it wasn't hard and didn't leave a mark, so I didn't bother reporting the incident". The patient appeared calm from an observational view during this clinical day.

Evidence-Based Approach

To render a solution, the problem must be evident through the reporting process to show that there is an increase of violence on medical floors and not just in the emergency room or mental health units. There are various factors that can lead to or induce workplace violence. The first would be a lack of an education program that would help staff point out cues of elevated stress level from the patient. Next would be the "perception that violence is tolerated, and reporting incidents will have no effect" (Occupational Safety and Health Administration [OSHA], n.d., p. 1). Finally, the understanding that if the violence is not reported than it did not happen (Arnetz et al., 2015). Ultimately, when the data is obtained, it will trigger the problem area that will assist with planning a course of action, followed by a solution.

Violence against healthcare workers is out-of-control. Recent statistics reveal that 62% percent of nurses nationwide reported that they have been verbally and physically attacked by patients; where approximately 42 percent reported the violent occurrence and of those that reported, 48 percent were not satisfied with the outcome or the way it was handled (American Nurses Association [ANA], 2018; Bolvin, 2018). Another study reveals that "80 percent of serious reported incidents happen in healthcare settings and caused by interactions with patients" (Occupational Safety and Health Administration [OSHA], 2015, p. 2).

Internal

If nurses were reporting all violent occurrences, there would be more accurate data to obtain of this epidemic. Due to the lack of reporting, one of the internal and evolving issues would be the morale and belief system that the organization will acknowledge or change a growing problem. There are different methods of reporting that can seem convoluted to understand as verbal reporting is not making it to paper or computer generated to see the data.

1) Verbal reporting to the next shift, charge nurse or nurse manager does not translate automatically to paper.
2) Nurses are not encouraged to report (Hogarth, Beattie, & Morphet, 2015).
3) The computer charting system may be unclear and does not offer a short form for reporting verbal and minor workplace violence incidences.
4) Workplace violence links are not on the computer software for reporting incidences, all workplace violence episodes go under miscellaneous and missed.
5) Nurses feel that the incident was not bad enough to warrant a report, as the violence is to be expected and a part of the job (Sofield & Salmond, 2003; Arnetz et al., 2015).

External

There are a couple external evolving issues that could be a direct or indirect contributor to the increased violence. The baseline education frameworks for both the practical and professional nursing curriculum does not outline more education on acute mental health or addiction (Florida Department of Education [FLDOE], 2018). Unless the nurse works in the emergency department or a mental health unit, then there will be additional training to help the nurse prevent or decrease escalation or injury. The health population and socioeconomic demographic of the area around the healthcare facility could be the other contributor to the increase of workplace violence. The Occupational Safety and Health Administration reported that the result of injuries sustained by a violent attack, reported or not reported could result in the nurse taking time off from work (Occupational Safety and Health Administration [OSHA], 2015). Which could lead to turnover with staff, poor staffing, low morale and poor job satisfaction scores. Ultimately affecting the bottom line of the organization, especially if they are not keeping current with population trends.

Every organization has their own interpretation of how they should handle the increase violence in the workplace. Some incorporated a workplace violence policy involving patient on nurse violence and education programs, some still have not. It is up to every leader that responds or observing my discussion post to reach out and make a difference in their organization. This is a huge gap in every system that depends on us to fix it. There has a bill has just been introduced but has not been passed, as it will be years before safeguards will be in place from a legislative level. In order to create a significant change in the healthcare setting, there needs to be active involvement from the organization's management team, which starts from the President of the company, all the way to the those working hands-on with the patient. If the culture remains the way it is right now, more nurses will be leaving the floor by leaving the profession or advancing their degree.

Change Proposal

To make a proposal for change, one has to think about what the best option is besides picking up a picketing sign and lose money by not working, fighting for a cause. Thinking logically and working towards a terminal degree over the last two-years, I have gained knowledge and expertise in this matter, personally, academically and professionally. I have gained credibility and a stance that allows me to discuss this challenge that others have and will hopefully not cringe away from in the coming months to years. The shift beyond the initial focus has already shown itself and revealed that nurses are not infallible. As we have all heard the circle of violence? We are not immune and how I believe is why lateral violence has increased as well. The learner must be ready and accepting for the change or the change will not happen.

Stakeholder involvement that are working within a certain target area is vital when creating goals and objectives when developing goals and objectives for a given program. The project that I am working on involves therapeutic concepts blending psychology and nursing, to not only help nurses reduce escalation from patients but to recognize that other stressors with work can translate through body language. Thus, resulting in the patient modeling the same behavior. The research should be from someone that represents the target population, who is a nurse that is active and has experience with working with acute mental health patients, combined with an expert in psychology (Huye, Connell, Cook, Yadrick, & Zoellner, 2014). An easy example as nurses, when administration comes up with a new rule or protocol which is far-fetched from the unit reality. How does the administration know what is really happening, if there is not data for support? They do not have a clue, unless a representative from the unit, maybe the unit manager, that can give updates, trends, and valuable information to help develop goals and objectives for a proposed program. Involving the target population, which in this case are nurses, may be a challenge as nurses are stressed, and some are even burned-out from working without support (Laeeque, Bilal, Babar, Khan, & Rahman, 2017). The one thing that I have observed over the years is if the nurse shows attitude on the unit, it can either create a hostile environment for other staff or even impede patient healing.

Resistance could be a factor; however, one could never know unless they try. One of the methods or approaches that I am using is holding a free event series targeted at helping nurses to decompress, talk about the issues that are affecting them, and how we as a nursing community can decrease patient verbal and physical escalation. Nurses like to vent through discussion, eating, sometimes exercising, and laughing. One of my goals is to let them do 2 of the four things, vent and laugh. We are a rare breed of individuals and with input from different nurses, over a period of the next 3 events, it is only the beginning to create a social change wave in nursing.

The aim is to facilitate the conversation by providing empathy to the nurse that is speaking and others that are attending. As the result, being the facilitator, this will help gather pertinent information about how the nurse is feeling, offer support, and in return, the nurse will model my behavior in their practice. What is the nurse's belief about taking care of the next mental health patient being admitted to their assignment? One method to change attitudes about mental health stigma and evaluating one's personal behavior, and how it can affect the outcome of someone suffering (Hodges & Videto, 2011). Influencing social change can also be through "increasing the motivation to comply with positive social pressure" (Hodges & Videto, 2011, p. 183). If the nurse participant does not like the event, there will not be a loss, as it was free, and the information will benefit nurses. They may even refer others to come, and if they come for round two in November, great! The goal of my practicum project is to receive information, model empathetic behavior, offer support, and help build up the profession that I love.

Chapter 9

Planning for Change

Violence in healthcare is growing out of control and the time is now to make a historic change. With the latest poll in 2018, the American Nurses Association has identified that "62% of nurses have personally experienced physical and verbal abuse on the job" (McClendon, Farbman, & Cipriano, 2018, para. 3). The numbers have sparked a movement called the End Nurse Abuse campaign, which starts in May and was chosen to be on the advisory panel. A few days after finding out the news, the Joint Commission released a sentinel event discussing the everyday violent occurrences that happen in the healthcare setting. The focus is in line with the first leg of the project, reporting barriers with the patient on nurse abuse. The plan is to create the culture of reporting, and safety of the units.

The root of the problem of physical and verbal abuse that has taken place has been accepted as a part of the job. Through several meetings with the nurses and various other support staff, it is evident through statements and body language that they are interested in making a difference with changing the environment. The root of creating change is through understanding the problem that is being presented. In this case, finding out how the nurses are feeling, not from my own experience but the common consensus. The plan is geared towards education of the current situation, national statistics, laws, facility policies, the evolution of patients to current, and the nursing behaviors towards reporting.

The current culture in the healthcare organization is predominately a "zero tolerance" to both patients and staff. However, the policy is usually one-sided, and nurses have reported that "nothing will be done anyway" (The Joint Commission, 2018). The other common statement among the nurses and nursing staff is that retaliation is a key factor to why reporting does not happen. It was further explained that worker's compensation pays roughly 60% of wages if there is no light duty available, which is rare if there is any. To subsidize their income from worker's compensation, their personal time off that was earned is mandated to be used when off from work. To sum up the issue at hand, nurses receive an injury on the unit or verbally abused, if they report it they are retaliated against by not only their employer but have a feeling of no support from their immediate leadership (Copeland & Henry, 2017). The other major finding was the policy that lays out the procedure for reporting the incidents to the charge nurse, nurse manager and then to the administrator on duty. If a violent code is called, then a report is filled out by the administrator on duty, or from the nurse themselves on the computerized charting system. The report that the nurse victim reports are not counted, there is no data to retrieve. The violent codes are counted, and they are minimal on average. Also, it is hard to find in the computerized charting system to report and have to enter it in as a different report, which takes approximately 10-15 minutes to complete on top of the nurses' existing assignment.

    The benefit outweighs the risk of implementing changes to protect nurses in the healthcare environment. When considering the stakeholders and end users, the loss of revenue and image is at the forefront. It costs the facility approximately "$27,000 to 103,000 in advertising, recruiting, hiring, orientation, and training" (Occupational Safety and Health Administration [OSHA], n.d., p. 4). Since the organization is a non-profit hospital system, in Florida the reimbursement is approximate "$2,224 per patient" (Rappleye, 2015, p. 2). Added together over 365 days, the total for one patient in a basic hospital unit with no intervention would equate to $811,760 per year. The small to average hospital holds approximately 80 patients, times it by $811,760 equates to $64,940,800 the hospital makes per year minus expenses. If the hospital loses 20 nurses per year, to find, hire, and train the new nurse, the hospital loses $2,060,000. The cost is minimal to what they make as a baseline, but this does not include other expenses incurred in running the facility. It is more cost effective to train and have safeguards in place to assist the nurses, for a safe working environment than to continuously hire new staff.

Implementing EBP Projects

Outcomes for the project are simple. To foster the development and growth of the culture of safety, with reporting incidents without retaliation, and ease of the process for nurses and nursing staff to report. Once the numbers are achieved, safeguards can go into place that involves acuity staffing, regulations, protections, and support systems for nursing staff. The outcome is reducing burn-out, post-traumatic stress disorder (PTSD), increase job satisfaction which will result in nursing retention. At the macro level, the current workplace violence policy does not enforce the "zero tolerance" criteria; it is geared more towards lateral violence versus patient on nurse abuse. If the department is found to have a high amount of violent codes called, then the organization will offer the healthcare workers the aggressive management training," if they are in behavioral health and extended to emergency room staff. The current practice is the AOD is recording the violent code data, the rest of the reported data is not being captured to pull for reference. On the micro level, patients have been at the forefront of satisfaction surveys that nursing turnover and one of the largest reasons why have been swept under the rug per say. Patient on nurse violence is a large component, in combination with unreported injuries, poor acuity staffing ratios, and the lack of resources to help nurses to feel empowered. To further compound the problem, nurses are either afraid to report the problem or believe that it is a "job norm" to be hurt by patients.

The most challenging part of the project is breaking through the adapted nursing behaviors and creating a culture of reporting. The goal of implementing this leg of the project is to discuss and educate the nurses that work on the unit, about the importance of reporting. By starting a dialog about reporting, nurses can express their concerns, personal attacks, and suggestions. When creating the system of reporting, the goal was simple. Keep it short and to the point. My preceptor found a locked box with a small opening for papers or tickets to go in. From that idea, I created small ballots that are short and simple to fill out. During the first meeting, the nurses start opening about how bad it can be on the floor and that patient on nurse violence is a norm on the unit. Because of the dialog, it had started the conversation that reporting the issue will positively result in the improvements of safety on the unit.

Evaluating the EBP Project

There are a couple of evaluation strategies that can be implemented to measure the effectiveness of the project. The first would include the growing interest from the nurses on the floor and ongoing conversation. Second would involve the balloting system, and the count of how many are reporting the incidents that are occurring. To create a culture, the momentum and interest have to be fostered through discussion with consistency. The new practice guideline is based on the results from the ballots and creating the ongoing conversation about the importance of reporting incidents. The new standard of safety would include reconfiguring the acuity to staffing ratios, enforce the zero-tolerance policy that is currently in place with amendments reflecting consequences for patients that injure or threaten nursing staff. The other addition should also include a teaching plan and therapeutic intervention for nurses that are traumatized.

Current State of Violence in Healthcare

The incidence of patient on nurse violence is growing at an epidemic rate. In April 2018, the Joint Commission release a sentinel event regarding the increase of patient on nurse violence and for places of employment to recognize and acknowledge the violence towards healthcare workers (The Joint Commission, 2018). A couple days later, the American Nurses Association acknowledged the sentinel event and stated that 62% of nurses stated that they were both verbally and physically injured while caring for patients (American Nurses Association [ANA], 2018). As a result, the End Nurse Abuse Advisory Panel was created, and I was a chosen to serve. With the statistics in mind, during this rotation, it was important to see if there were any changes being implemented within my current clinical situation. Currently, there is not a plan in place to work with nurses to help decrease escalation or assist with coping mechanisms. Using the examples of past clinical rotations and what I am observing at the other clinical site, is the non-verbal communication. One area of observation is the repetitive actions from the nurse, with completing shift tasks and the interaction they are having with the patient. Is the nurse engaged in conversation with the patient? Are they smiling and portraying positive body language, exhibiting eye contact, and smiling? Within reason, verbal communication will also be scrutinized as it also plays a vital role in the patient care experience. Communication is important to watch for, as key components of providing a positive patient experience, and maintaining a safe work environment.

When applying a theory to patient on nurse violence, it is resiliency that allows nurses to care for their 5-7 patient assignment, become injured or get yelled at by a family member then wipe their tears and move on (Polk, 1997). The problem of nurses not having the ability to recoup from both verbal and physical altercations can begin the process of burn-out (Zysk, 2018). The goal of this practicum is to find possible barriers that could create miscommunication and the beginning of behavior escalation. My role as a doctoral student is to observe the workflow, communication between nurses and patients, create a helpful education plan targeting communication, and evaluate the nurse's response if it was helpful in their practice. I am looking forward to the results, as this will be completed through the monthly events and through clinical experience.

Nonverbal Behavior Awareness in Nurses

Problem statement:

Will helping nurses to recognize nonverbal communication, reduce the number of patient escalation events?

The population targeted in this phase of program planning are those who have mental illness and addiction issues. Over the last few years there, has been an increased awareness of patients that have attacked nurses on health care units. The most recent poll conducted in April 2018 from the American Nurses Association, states that 62 percent of nurses across the United

States has admitted to being verbally and physically attacked (American Nurses Association [ANA], 2018). The Joint Commission had also released a Sentinel Event Alert stating that "each episode of violence or credible threat to health care workers" (The Joint Commission, 2018, para. 3). When thinking back to several witnessed attacks on nurses, there were crucial behaviors that were noticed in almost every situation.

The nurse was stressed out, had a full assignment of roughly 5-7 patients, that was not triaged according to their illness for a fair patient assignment. Most recently, a nurse was caring for three addicted and withdrawing patients that had some form of mental illness on a medical-surgical floor, along with two that were admitted for post-surgical intervention and observation. This nurse was not communicating effectively both verbally or physically. The nurse was observed rolling her eyes and smirking at the patient while they were trying to tell her they were in pain. What the nurse was saying sounded direct but kind. Other times, nurses would look in on their patients and if the nurse was stopped for a question, the nurse would sigh or even say they would be back and never show. All the while, the patient has a possibility of feeling neglected or not important to the nurse.

Chapter 10

Identifying a Theory

In the world of being a nurse, who would have thought that psychology and nursing were not as intertwined as they should be. Identifying the best theory to apply to this practicum project is essential, to take a closer look with taking into consideration current societal trends and what is happening on health care units. It is a regular occurrence in the mid-western Florida region to have approximately 3-4 acute mental health or addiction patients. When you consider the level of education that is taught for acute mental health and addiction in nursing school, it amounts to a week of theory and maybe a clinical rotation or two. In the nursing profession, it is vital to start blending psychology with nursing, not only for our patients but as professionals that are trying to help others reach optimal health.

The first theorist is Jean Watson's theory of caring; this is the go-to theory for nursing. As nurses, we have identified the power of connection, as it is important when you are caring for every patient. When caring for oneself, nurses have issues in this area. There are many aspects have changed over the years in nursing which has shifted to not only a personal self-care deficit but increased stress levels. The patient population has evolved, where the nursing curriculum and training have not, leaving nurses vulnerable to care for oneself, hoping that the employer will provide safety and security to do their job. Looking at Florida statistics from 2016, the medical examiner noted that St. Petersburg is the second hardest hit with prescription overdose deaths in Florida (Florida Department of Law Enforcement, 2017). When a nurse has not worked with mental health or addiction patients, they tend to treat and think all patients are the same, especially since they are on a medical-surgical or even working in labor and delivery. The patient does not have to be categorized and placed on a mental health floor for a broken leg.

Albert Bandura's social cognitive theory is the best fit for nurses that are academically unprepared to work under stressful circumstances. When a nurse is rushing around caring for actively withdrawing patients, those with medical conditions, or on suicide watch can become challenging to handle when the acuity does not match the staffing grid. The nurse may also have an underlying mental health issue that could be diagnosed or undiagnosed that could lead to inappropriate responses or body language, including facial expressions. What Bandura's theory focused on was not only of a person's belief in their capabilities but how stress and depression that one feels can become taxing on a person, creating a negative situation (Bandura, 1989).

The best example is when a nurse has two patients that are simultaneously withdrawing, the patient calls the nurse in for the fifth time and says they are in pain and need medication now. One of the symptoms of opioid withdraw is body aches. Instead the nurse's face turns red and rolls her eyes. As a result, the patient observing the nurse's response resulting in an elevated reaction from the patient. Time passes by, the nurse said that she would be back, the patient calls again, but even more upset. The patient is scoring high on the opioid withdraw scoring sheet, but the nurse did not know to do it. The patient begins to escalate as they are suffering and asking for help. Through observation, the patient felt they could simulate and increase their behavior over the nurse's, so the nurse would know that the patient is suffering and needs help.

Literature Review

There is an abundance of information about patient on nurse violence, even reporting barriers. The problem of patient on nurse violence is prevalent and widespread in the literature obtained. Two articles that stand out discusses the harmful effects of healthcare units regarding violent acts against nurses and burnout syndrome. The result of escalation must involve more than just the patient being entirely at fault and irrational, as for every action receives a reaction. The first article points out that the escalation could be a result of something the nurse may have done to provoke the patient, either directly or indirectly (Chen, Huang, Hwang, & Chen, 2010). Second article discusses how stress over a long period of time can induce burn-out among nurses through high-emotional exhaustion, feelings of professional underachievement, and depersonalization (Ribeiro et al., 2014, p. 4). Nurses may or may not realize that what we think could portray in our facial expressions and actions. Finding the missing piece could help create a program to help nurses with understanding that it is not all what we say, it is also how we say it. When putting this observation into the mix of patient on nurse abuse, it cannot be discounted that nonverbal communication could be a proponent of the problem.

Needs Assessment

There are different approaches for gathering information on a particular need of a population. Physical observation of interactions, primary data collection from research, and interviewing the nurses on the units are the methods used for gathering information on person to person interactions. Through self-expression of stress, observation of the nurse running around trying to take care of their patients, while juggling call lights, and passing medication, what the nurse would frequently state how they have not had a lunch, gone to the bathroom or even taken a 15-minute break just to sit down. Frequently, the shifts would be 12 hours and at times, the nurses will be asked to work longer to cover someone that called in for their shift. The basic needs according to Maslow's Hierarchy of Needs are often unmet, which could be a potential challenge and a factor leading to adverse non-verbal communication.

One of the easiest solutions to propose is to make break time mandatory, where the nurse is made to take their uninterrupted lunch, without their work phone. Not only the nurse will have something to eat but they will have a recharge to keep hustling with their assignment. More needs to happen, but the first step is ensuring that the basic needs are met. The next challenge is the nurse may not be willing to self-reflect as they often relate their lack of administration support to the challenges they face on the unit. Leading to the need for safety and security, where the nurse is faced with unsafe working conditions and often understaffed (DeMarco & Tilson, n.d.). Lastly, the nurse may also have an underlying mental health condition that they may or may not be diagnosed or treated. Compounding the increase level of stress with a mental health issue, the nurse may begin to feel overwhelmed, leading to burn-out and possibly post-traumatic stress disorder (PTSD) (Mealer, Burnham, Goode, Rothbaum, & Moss, 2009). All nurses are trained according to medical needs and therapies, unless specializing, they are unaware of how to work with those that are suffering from a mental illness. The proposed remedy is to help nurses learn more about what they can do at the moment to decrease patient escalation. The goal is to be present and employ active listening, as most patients cannot help their actions, and many could be reciprocating the behavior they observe.

Communication

As previously noted, the plan was to observe primarily non-verbal communication, where since then, the project focus has been reverted to both verbal and non-verbal communication. The observation in the field has been interesting which has helped to open the practicum experience from just a small office setting and past experiences. When out in a clinical setting, observations include the flow of the unit during care and the behaviors from staff or the patient during the practicum day. Insights gained include the increased workload and how it can indirectly overwhelm a nurse who may have patients that are over acuity and difficult to manage. One of the main reasons is the lack of education and policies about working with those suffering from mental illness or addiction (Occupational Safety and Health Administration [OSHA], 2015). With the increase of violence occurring in the emergency department, there is a likelihood that these violent patients are being admitted to varying units in the hospital where training is not offered (Gacki-Smith et al., 2009). Research methods of how to facilitate professional growth through therapeutic communication and redirect negative comments or responses.

The last few weeks have set forth a huge barrier, and that is nurses not taking to the notion that they may be a contributor to the violence being ensued. In the clinical setting, the enemy is mainly administration when it comes to why the assignments and functionality are not working and all the reason why nurses are being injured. The reality is that the nursing curriculum for both the practical and professional nursing programs contain minimal mental health training, leaving the nursing profession vulnerable to increased violence (Florida Department of Education [FLDOE], 2018). The goal is to continue promoting the free events to help inform nurses of simple ways to keep or foster the nurse/patient relationship and create a culture of safety.

One of the pieces when developing the education that stood out, was the increase of awareness of violence against nurses with just the American Nurses Association and decided to share with the audience the difference of focus between 2017 and 2018 with underreporting unit violence (Bolvin, 2018). If the workplace violence incident is not reported, then it never happened, resulting in more of the same incidences on the units. Until legislation is passed for protection against violent occurrences, an education plan is needed to help nurses increase therapeutic communication techniques to decrease incidences and increase job satisfaction. The goal for change is to continue being vigilant and work with nurses that are accepting of the training. If the administration team joined in and supported the training effort, the education plan will be more effective and help open avenues, increasing the likelihood of change occurring. It is an on-going issue with more experienced nurses joining in on the discussion due to feelings of "nothing being done, and that violence is a part of the job" (Gacki-Smith et al., 2009). The unit goal would be to incorporate role-playing exercises to help nurses feel more comfortable when working with those suffering from mental illness and addiction.

I decided to perform a mini experiment along with the therapeutic communication techniques. The goal was to introduce smiling more into the equation with actively listening to the patient. Most communication methods in a stressful environment in the workplace, can appear more transactional, and the perception from the patient is the nurse is not paying attention or listening to their concerns (Wienclaw, 2017). Nonverbal and verbal communication can translate into a misunderstanding when a patient is not feeling well. By changing how we perceive ourselves in this process, can greatly affect our relationship with the patient as what we say or do may be misinterpreted. Gathering this information was crucial to this project.

Winding down from a very busy but a productive quarter, the information gathered and observed among nurses was a pivotal point with the progress of the project. The stakeholders involved in this project, nurses, realized that making a simple adjustment of changing their nonverbal gestures and increasing their therapeutic communication, helped when working with patients. The interactions went from a making a transaction, such as a nursing assessment or passing medications to building a relationship with the patient, which resulted in less behavior escalation episodes from patients this quarter.

When aligning a concept such as how nonverbal communication could affect the patient-nurse relationship, it is important to consider what will help the learning program or impede growth. The stakeholder, or audience, for this program, would be nurses that work with patients in a healthcare setting, the environment (Hodges & Videto, 2011). Benefits for the stakeholder by learning the program, includes recognizing the nonverbal communication that may contribute to patient behavior escalation. The second is through awareness, the stakeholder could create a patient-nurse relationship by being present physically in the patient's care, creating a calmer environment. For example, instead of sitting at the nurse's station, to sit closer to the patient room, even outside their door if they are having signs or symptoms of anxiety. Of course, if the patient is visibly anxious, to see if they have something ordered. Actions with patients suffering from mental illness is important. These actions could be listening, staying close to the patient, following through on statements, open body language, and eye contact (Brent, 2016).

The challenge is great for introducing this concept and finding nursing participants to have an open mind, regarding possible behavior changes. Many nurses are overworked, upset, tired, frustrated, understaffed, injured, and frankly do not care to hear that they have done anything wrong. It is important to understand this as there may be nurses that are watching the progression and eventually may participate. As for finding the facility that would assist in adopting the program, they may use the program but introduce it in a punitive manner, not in an objective or non-persecutory manner. The goal for introducing the program is to see the intermediate progress, which shows the decrease of escalation and the final outcome, increasing job satisfaction with nurses when working with challenging patients or situations (Kettner, Moroney, & Martin, 2017).

One of the strategies for overcoming barriers is to request and listen to the nurse participants, modeling the behavior that is the goal of teaching the program. It is important to be the example of how nurses should behave when patients are distressed. For example, as the nurse is discussing their experience and releasing their stress or feelings about a situation that happened to them, they will see that venting is not only therapeutic, but it is showing them that this is what the patient is doing. Working as the scenario of I am them on the floor with the upset patient venting to me. It is not personal; they are just going through something bigger than us. The barrier to the program design, would be the automatic acceptance of implementing it into practice and personal perception from the administration.

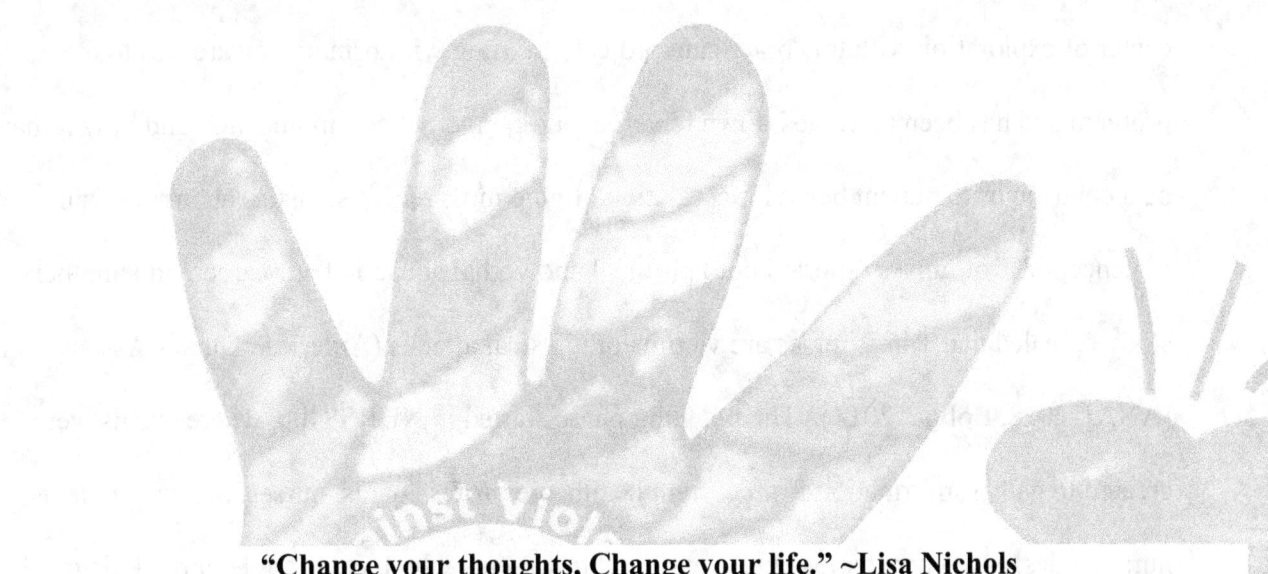

"Change your thoughts, Change your life." ~Lisa Nichols

Chapter 11

Planning for the Practicum

The rise of patient on nurse verbal and physical violence in healthcare settings is the center of exploration with this practicum project. Starting with bringing awareness to the problem and has been narrowed down to verbal and nonverbal communication and how it may be a contributor to patient behavior escalation. In the most recent statistics about the rising violence, 62% of nurses reported both physical and verbal abuse in their career, and another study revealed that 1 in 5 nurses are victims of physical attacks (American Nurses Association [ANA], 2018; Bolvin, 2018). The planning phase started in NURS8400, where events were created to gather information from current healthcare professionals, nurses, nursing students, nurses aides, and others exposed to working with patients who have a single or dual diagnosis of addiction and mental health. One of the identified sources to the problem was a lack of mental health and addiction training in the frameworks for the Florida nursing curriculum (Florida Department of Education [FLDOE], 2018). At the school where I currently teach the practical nursing program, a standard curriculum is not in place for all nursing instructors. Each nurse creates their curriculum and adheres to how many hours allotted for the subject taught. As a result, this may not allow much time or allow for the nursing instructor to recover material and resources for the section if they are not proficient or specialized. The goal for this practicum project is to help nurses find satisfaction in their nursing career, to love what they do and know how to work with patients that have possible social challenges or processing issues.

Learning Objectives

1) Understand how the increase in work demands that could increase the likelihood of increasing patient escalation.

2) Analyze the types of interactions that nurses are having with patients.

3) Create an education program that will help the nurse to increase interpersonal interactions versus transactional.

1) Assess the impact of the training program with patient and nurse's interactions on the unit.

The planning and implementation of this practicum project have shifted slightly as the focus is mainly set to recognize the systematic transactions and how a decrease of interpersonal relationships with the patient could increase behavior escalation (Armstrong, 2017). With the growing number of responsibilities that nurses are expected to juggle, nurses are so busy that they might not realize how their body language or how incorporating more active listening into their daily routine could make their shift virtually behavior free ("Effective Listening," 2018). The combination of the patient that may have underlying mental illness, compounded with the fear of the unknown or otherwise known as situational anxiety may not mix well with the overwhelmed nurse's reactions. When the patient is admitted for unknown medical diagnosis, they will be fearful to a degree, as they are unsure what it is happening and in an unfamiliar setting or environment (Jaruzel & Gregoski, 2017).

Another example, if the patient is admitted involuntarily for a psychiatric hold for safety concerns, the patient may be on a heightened amount of anxiety and may interpret the nurse's actions to be undesirable. As a result, the patient may escalate. Creating an education plan will focus on assisting nurses in how they can help prevent verbal and physical violence towards not only themselves, to other patients, but also co-workers. Lastly, to evaluate how the education plan touched on areas in need of improvement. The goal is to re-evaluate and ensure the last leg of the project, I will be a substantial and executable practicum project. Key leadership activities include, but not limited to the initiative of conducting free events for nurses to not only network but come together for support, facilitate a conversation about bringing positive change within the nursing community, and learn how to incorporate active listing skills into their practice. The goal for this project is to help the nurse to feel empowered, not overwhelmed, and satisfied with the care given to their patients during the shift. Ultimately, the patient will feel more relaxed, have an uninterrupted healing process, and be discharged when stable.

Observed activity

The objectives of this rotation set are to:

Analyze and dissect the current information about the ease of reporting procedures.

Evaluate the learner's understanding about reporting procedures.

Create an educational forum to improve understanding about reporting procedures with an increase in workplace violence reporting by May 1st.

Throughout the practicum experience, there was ongoing dialog about the importance of reporting workplace violence. While analyzing the current method of reporting, it was apparent that the reporting system is lengthy, hard to navigate, and not conducive for reporting workplace violence. While on the unit, the goal was to evaluate the learner's understanding about reporting incidents. The behavior of the nurse was being kicked, slapped, and spit on was the norm of nursing. Reporting started to dwindle after the month of being on the floor. When working with the nurses, the goal was to create a culture of reporting and recognizing what happens if the patient is not reported. The resistance of "nothing will change" continued.

Implementing an Educational Forum

Creating the educational forum was a segment to reiterate the importance of reporting, but to also understand the behavior of the patient and how the nurse unknowingly contributes to the escalation that the current culture has cultivated from the organizational level. It was difficult to not be blunt and tell the staff about the reporting holes, so the goal was to not penalize and remain professional, while educating the nurses about what happens the escalation is not reported. The nurses, all with an Associates to having their Doctor of Nursing Practice, did not put two thoughts together about not reporting the incident, that it was virtually a permission of sorts for the patient to continue the bad behavior. When one nurse stated that she has reported the incident to her charge nurse, that was a positive indication that nurses are trying to report but the follow through and data capture is not there. By the end of the forum, the nurses appeared satisfied and thanked me for the insight and knowledge about the importance of reporting. After the educational forum, my preceptor wanted me to take the information and scheduled a meeting for me to come in and speak with all the educators and nurse managers in the facility to extend the reporting piece of the project. The day before this was to take place, I received a call stating that I was not able to finish my rotation, despite already completing the practicum hours and this would have been voluntary. The explanation was that since I was not an employee anymore, that

I would not be able to complete the rotations. The university was pushing for a letter from their legal department for acceptance, especially since I had previously completed a master's with the organization, the goal was that it would be a benefit to help them. After I completed the hours in the system, my preceptor stated that she looks forward to reading about the progress of changing the nursing culture and wished me well. It was a sad day for me as we were making progress in achieving a safer environment for the nursing staff and patients.

When you feel like giving up..Just Remember – It takes just one rock to start the rippling effect of change. ~Dr. Sandy

Chapter 12

Not-So-Modern Nursing Education

The magnitude of patient on nurse violence is not only detrimental to the profession but opens a conversation about translating evidence to a solution. In recent statistics, 62% of nurses have been cursed at, threatened, spit on, punched, or stabbed with a weapon while performing their job functions (American Nurses Association [ANA], 2018). With the overwhelming amount of injuries and compounded anxiety, many nurses have developed burn-out, post-traumatic stress disorder (PTSD), and a decrease of compassion satisfaction (Schmidt & Haglund, 2017). Observations throughout my nursing career and recent times, there has been a shift in patient population that the nursing curriculum frameworks does not fully address. According to the latest statistics, "44.7 million people" which equates to "one in five U.S. adults" lives with a mental illness, with 19.2 million (43.1%) sought mental health treatment (National Institute of Mental Health, 2017, para. 1). Approximately "22.5 million people, over 12 years old, self-reported that they needed treatment with their substance abuse, and 11.8 million adults stated that they needed mental health treatment" (Substance Abuse and Mental Health Services Administration [SAMHSA], 2018, para. 2).

As the "fee for service" approaches an end of its lifecycle, facilities will no longer receive payment for errors and preventable events (White, Dudley-Brown, & Terhaar, 2016, p. 115). Insights from theory has help guide and narrow down the focus of the practicum problem to relationship building instead of focus on just the problem itself of patients attacking nursing staff. Changes that are underway begin with finding the source, questioning why patients are escalating. What is happening that is causing a patient to get upset? What is the patient is the patient upset about? What is the patient/nurse ratio? These are just a few questions that should be considered when discovering to root of the problem. Literature has also suggested the need for increase an anti-violence training for nurses, as it helps nurses to work with those that are potentially volatile (Zhao et al., 2015). The point that is crucial to make is that not even the pre-nursing frameworks suggest an increase of mental health, to help those in a nursing program to know how to communicate with patients, understand self-care and how we interact with patients can increase the outcome of violence.

Implementing change starts with assessing the nurse learner's knowledge about communication, their desire to learn new information, and experiences which they may share with unit challenges. At that point, facilitating a conversation about why patients may escalate, guiding the conversation about what nurses could do in our own practice to help the patient to have a healing experience. That our job as a nurse is to not judge, but to carry out the plan of care for our patients. As a leader, it is important to build the desired interpersonal relationships along with exhibiting positive nonverbal and verbal open communication with the nursing staff. Teaching by example, is the best way to duplicate behavior. Throughout the day, nurses are systematically assessing their patients, giving medications, talking with doctors, and more times than not, the patient acuity is not balanced which increases the likelihood that not all patients are going to receive the same attention.

Helping the nurse to build a relationship with their patients will not only help them reduce the stress of juggling complicated patients but reduce their stress level. Most of the time, not in my personal nursing experience, I would purposely take the hardest and "most annoying patients" on my assignment per the nurse that would beg me to take them. More times than not, the therapeutic patient/nurse relationship would be prevalent though various positive interactions by listening, laugh with them and despite the repetition, when my shift was over, I was tired but not stressed out. Being a nurse's aide climbing the ranks, it is easier for other nurses to listen, especially new ones, as they aim to avoid the problems that nurses are facing because they are more prepared. The goal during practicum was to understand the increased workload, analyze the types of interactions nurses have with patients, create an education program to increase interpersonal relationships, and assess the impact of the training program with patient and nurse interactions.

Nursing School and Lack of Mental Health and Addiction Education

My experience on the floor for over 28 years, I have seen the violence not only increase from patients but have also seen my share of nurses that are suffering compassion fatigue. Nurses may not recognize the unintentional nonverbal or verbal communication connection that is linked with little mental health and addiction training that is learned in nursing school. Therefore, it could escalate the patient whether the nurse means to be cross with the patient or not, the patient may escalate. If the patient is suffering from addiction or severe mental illness, they may not comply with boundaries and triggered to become out of control (Colvin & Sugai, 1989).

When completing the doctoral scholarly project, it is important to explore every avenue of an outcome that contributes to the care of every individual. The Essential II: Organizational and systems leadership for quality improvement and systems thinking, has been determined to fit the criteria for this practicum (American Association of Colleges of Nursing [AACN], 2006). The goal is to investigate the current organizational policy and procedures to increase quality, find gaps or holes, and how the admission process could be improved. Information gathered will be a section in a three-part series to determine external sources, such as facility processes that could contribute to patient on nurse escalation, which could have been prevented.

Learning Objectives

1) Define the admission process for those suffering from addiction and acute mental health symptoms.
2) Examine the current policy, assess for a gap and need of education.
3) Demonstrate competency by developing a staff education plan that supports or enhances the current workplace violence policy.

Activities

1) Read the current policies and procedures for admission of those addicted and with acute mental illness.
    a. Time elapsed from entering the unit to admission to the floor.
        i. Medical clearance
    b. Baker Act system – When individuals are a harm to themselves or others (Department of Mental Health Law & Policy, 2014).
        i. Voluntary
        ii. Involuntary
        iii. Marchman Act

2) Assimilate the information and the policy that is currently in place.

   a. Zero-tolerance
      i. Lateral violence
      ii. Patient/Family violence
   b. Education
      i. Programs geared towards prevention.
         1. Prevention
         2. Codes
         3. De-escalation

3) Formulate recommendations and revisions of the policy with a short staff in-service of changes if the facility agrees to adopt updates. If not, create an in-service of facility policies that were previously adopted.

Timeline

The proposed timeline for this section is approximately ten-weeks, taking roughly two to three weeks per learning objective combined with the activity. During the admission process, it is important to observe the time it takes for the patient to receive medical clearance and admitted to a mental health unit. The next area to consider is if the patient is a Baker Act, what the patient may need for safety, or are they a valid hold. The policies and procedures for admission are detrimental to the plan of care so it is essential to know what they are and how to proceed with each area of care. Finally, in the last 2-3 weeks, a short education in-service will be developed with the existing prevention programs to enhance what is currently in place. If there is not a plan in place, it would be beneficial to work with nurses to learn how to respond to patients, prevent behavior codes, and if absolutely necessary, de-escalate. Finally, to offer a short educational in-service to enhance the facility's existing educational materials and training.

De-Escalation vs. Prevention Education

Due to the uncertainty and unforgiving task of working with patients and their family members that are equally imbalanced can not only create a hostile environment but can chew away at the morale of a new or experienced nurse. Workplace violence is becoming an epidemic where "40-75% of healthcare workers have reported suffering from verbal and physical abuse" (Cox, 2017, p. 2). The use of clinical reasoning is utilized through using both formal and informal ways of strategizing care for an irrational patient through obtaining their information, evaluating the circumstances for the behavior, and determine various actions to de-escalate or prevent the situation from occurring (Simmons, 2009). As nurses, we are faced with patients that are suffering from some form of mental illness throughout our bedside careers. Patients and their families are suffering from some form of anxiety, where it can render a person to fear the unknown. In combination with a mental health condition, it can create negative behavior that can result in violence on the unit. Another form of clinical reasoning is when the nurse uses their "knowledge in combination with clinical experiences" that identifies the possibility and avenues of escalation where escalation could begin (Lee, Lee, Bae, & Seo, 2016, p. 75).

P - Nurses

I - De-escalation techniques

C - Nurses not using the de-escalation techniques

O - Prevention of patient escalation

T - Admission to discharge

Research Question:

Does the incidence of violence against nurses decrease when de-escalation tactics are used?

When analyzing the latest statistics on violence against nurses, one could question if the institution is working to fix the problem or to provide and implement an education plan that may or may not be affective. The most recent statistics obtained from the Advisory Board states that "between 2011 and 2013, nearly 75% of all workplace assaults happen in healthcare, 80% of emergency medical workers experience physical violence, and only 13% of nurses report physical abuse" ("Workplace violence," 2016, para. 3). Failure to report these incidents tends to lesson the problem to the administration and those who pull institution data. The lack of reporting from the nursing staff has been an on-going issue as one does not want to be perceived as "weak among their peer, nobody was hurt", and that is a part of the job (Copeland & Henry, 2017, p. 71). This topic is of great interest to me, so it is an on-going conversation that I have with many nurses on the unit floors. Some employers have started de-escalation programs for those that become verbally and physically violent. My concerns are great with this kind of program, as it masks the problem and does not prevent the escalation. Most of the time poor acuity matching to the staffing ratios is the problem. Overloading a nurse is not the solution, but can be done by accident, as it is impossible to know all patients that flow through the hospital setting. The goal is to prevent the problem before the patient become belligerent and out of control.

Chapter 12

Collaboration and Accountability from Leadership

To have an efficient workflow, there must be collaboration from all sides and every party involved in the care of a patient. In addition to collaboration, it is vital that accountability from leaders is present to "meet the challenges and reduce error" within an organization and to provide support, regardless of their background (White, Dudley-Brown, & Terhaar, 2016, p. 115). As most nurses would agree, this is very rare when working on medical units. During one of the observations this quarter, it was apparent that administration stays in the office to maintain the appearance of the chain of command where the supervisor is either in meetings all day or avoided on the unit. One thing that I have learned over the years is that many leaders in an organization may or may not accept feedback, and most of the time as a staff nurse, I was often a target for lateral violence. However, there have been times where engaging the supervisor with peer support, often helped to build a case for improvements or protocol updates through shared governance. To be a leader that can exhibit effective interprofessional communication, is one that knows their own limitations, exhumes confidence in their skills and area of expertise, respecting culture, encourages insight, and encourages teamwork (Center, 2018).

Before implementing any sort of education program with nurses, the stakeholder, it is important to assess their current knowledge or concerns about their interactions with patients. During the daily routine, the nurse completes their assessments, passes medications, applies treatments, and performs activities of daily living. The focus of the practicum is primarily on building relationships with patients and preventing the feeling as if the situation or procedure occurring is transactional. With the results of the survey, observation of the patient and nurse interactions and create short in-services that target phases of how to build relationships, the nurse leader has the vital information to present for increased support with an education program. The in-service could incorporate other areas of the healthcare system, such as; admissions, pharmacy, appointment scheduling, and therapeutic services to provide an interprofessional collaborative approach. By having the collaborative support from the shared governance, surveys for data, and unit observations of various roles, approaching those with power and authority will appreciate the abundance of organized information and approve of the mini-series of in-services in efforts to bring up patient satisfaction scores.

Knowledge Integration and Communication

Integrating knowledge into everyday experiences and actions is vital to creating success for any medical unit or healthcare agency. One of the largest barriers in healthcare is the lack of communication and support from those not experiencing unit challenges firsthand (Homested, 2000). To assist in the resolution of unit challenges, is to track the surveys that patients leave for unit floors, in combination with feedback from the shared governance team. Then create an anonymous reporting system from floor nurses to report concerns the nurse have and hold weekly meetings to address and create a plan to correct the minor issue. If there is no resolve, the next step would be to include all avenues taken to resolve the issue and present to the supervisor. The supervisor and the shared governance team would be in communication about the unresolved issue and either create a plan or it may have to climb to the next level with the added support. Through an effective communication processes, the confidence, and gained trust from colleagues can be a huge benefit to the healthcare agency as it builds trust with prompt response or even changing the status quo (Center, 2018). The need for facility involvement in the process of change, can be a difficult feat and teach the doctoral student a few things about the importance of their project.

The incidence of patient on nurse violence is growing at an epidemic rate. In April 2018, the Joint Commission release a sentinel event regarding the increase of patient on nurse violence and for places of employment to recognize and acknowledge the violence towards healthcare workers (The Joint Commission, 2018). A couple days later, the American Nurses Association acknowledged the sentinel event and stated that 62% of nurses stated that they were both verbally and physically injured while caring for patients (American Nurses Association [ANA], 2018). As a result, the End Nurse Abuse Advisory Panel was created, and I was a chosen to serve. With the statistics in mind, during this rotation, it was important to see if there were any changes being implemented within my current clinical situation. Currently, there is not a plan in place to work with nurses to help decrease escalation or assist with coping mechanisms. Using the examples of past clinical rotations and what I am observing at the other clinical site, is the non-verbal communication. One area of observation is the repetitive actions from the nurse, with completing shift tasks and the interaction they are having with the patient. Is the nurse engaged in conversation with the patient? Are they smiling and portraying positive body language, exhibiting eye contact, and smiling? Within reason, verbal communication will also be scrutinized as it also plays a vital role in the patient care experience. Communication is important to watch for, as key components of providing a positive patient experience, and maintaining a safe work environment.

When applying a theory to patient on nurse violence, it is resiliency that allows nurses to care for their 5-7 patient assignment, become injured or get yelled at by a family member then wipe their tears and move on (Polk, 1997). The problem of nurses not having the ability to recoup from both verbal and physical altercations can begin the process of burn-out (Zysk, 2018). The goal of this practicum is to find possible barriers that could create miscommunication and the beginning of behavior escalation. My role as a doctoral student s to was to observe the workflow, communication between nurses and patients, create a helpful education plan targeting communication, and evaluate the nurse's response if it was helpful in their practice. I am looking forward to the results, as this will be completed through the monthly events and through clinical experience.

As previously noted, the plan was to observe primarily non-verbal communication, where since then, the project focus has been reverted to both verbal and non-verbal communication. The observation in the field has been interesting which has helped to open the practicum experience from just a small office setting and past experiences. When out in a clinical setting, observations include the flow of the unit during care and the behaviors from staff or the patient during the practicum day. Insights gained include the increased workload and how it can indirectly overwhelm a nurse who may have patients that are over acuity and difficult to manage. One of the main reasons is the lack of education and policies about working with those suffering from mental illness or addiction (Occupational Safety and Health Administration [OSHA],

2015). With the increase of violence occurring in the emergency department, there is a likelihood that these violent patients are being admitted to varying units in the hospital where training is not offered (Gacki-Smith et al., 2009). Research methods of how to facilitate professional growth through therapeutic communication and redirect negative comments or responses.

The last few weeks have set forth a huge barrier, and that is nurses not taking to the notion that they may be a contributor to the violence being ensued. In the clinical setting, the perceived enemy is mainly administration when it comes to why the assignments and functionality are not working and all the reason why nurses are being injured. The reality is that the nursing curriculum for both the practical and professional nursing programs contain minimal mental health training, leaving the nursing profession vulnerable to increased violence (Florida Department of Education [FLDOE], 2018). The goal is to continue promoting the free events to help inform nurses of simple ways to keep or foster the nurse/patient relationship and create a culture of safety. One of the pieces when developing the education that stood out, was the increase of awareness of violence against nurses with just the American Nurses Association and decided to share with the audience the difference of focus between 2017 and 2018 with underreporting unit violence (Bolvin, 2018). If the workplace violence incident is not reported, then it never happened, resulting in more of the same incidences on the units. Until legislation is passed for protection against violent occurrences, an education plan is needed to help nurses increase therapeutic communication techniques to decrease incidences and increase job satisfaction.

The goal for change is to continue being vigilant and work with nurses that are accepting of the training. If the administration team joined in and supported the training effort, the education plan will be more effective and help open avenues, increasing the likelihood of change occurring. It is an on-going issue with more experienced nurses joining in on the discussion due to feelings of "nothing being done, and that violence is a part of the job" (Gacki-Smith et al., 2009). The unit goal would be to incorporate role-playing exercises to help nurses feel more comfortable when working with those suffering from mental illness and addiction.

Winding down from a very busy but a productive quarter, the information gathered and observed among nurses was a pivotal point with the progress of the project. The stakeholders involved in this project, nurses, realized that making a simple adjustment of changing their nonverbal gestures and increasing their therapeutic communication, helped when working with patients. The interactions went from a making a transaction, such as a nursing assessment or passing medications to building a relationship with the patient, which resulted in less behavior escalation episodes from patients this quarter.

Application of Clinical Reasoning

The application of clinical reasoning should involve various forms of learning. The first would include the breaking down information that can be used to or enhance critical thinking during behavior escalation. Recalling the previous event and how that turned out and what could have been done differently to prevent the escalation. Next would include a simulation program that will interact with the learner to provoke thought with scenarios, and progress into more violent code situations. Finally, it is the "nurse's responsibility to accurately interpret the human responses, to select the appropriate intervention" with a viable outcome (De Carvalho, Oliveiro-Kumakura, & Vasconcelos Morais, 2016, p. 663). The refinement of the evidence-based project question would have to include recalling previous behavior issues, and attribute factors leading up to the escalation of behavior. In addition to recalling the scenarios and the combination of evidence-based research, it will assist into a plan and "strategy for action" (Terry, 2018, p. 16).

The focus of this rotation is to continue implementing the educational program, evaluate the effectiveness of the learned material from the stakeholders, and disseminate the information as a final project for this practicum. During the re-evaluation phase of the last practicum, I met with my preceptor to discuss where we left off and where I see the remainder of the project going for this final phase. We discussed the different areas previously covered, including the relationship between patients and nurses, verbal and non-verbal communication techniques to decrease patient on nurse violence, and coping mechanisms. This rotation will continue to focus on the nurse-patient relationship. The goal is to analyze how external stimuli and an increased patient workload can affect morale, the strain on nurses to perform for the organization, which can directly or indirectly result in verbal and physical abuse from patients (Fasanya & Dada, 2015). The essentials were adjusted to precisely align the objectives throughout the project.

It is important to continue researching and recalling previous information to incorporate into this final rotation. The goal was to find environmental factors that could bring about negative behavior in both nurse and patient. A few areas right away observed was the lighting, call bells, telemetry monitors, intravenous medication pumps, and the noise of conversations being held at the nurse's station. While standing for a few minutes observing the workflow, you can hear gossip and snarky comments about the prior shift. There was another episode where a nurse made comments of the night shift having it "easy as they did not have all of the responsibilities they did on days." The discussions on the unit between staff were minimal, but there were also nonverbal eye-rolling and dirty looks when asked to help another nurse out in a crunch situation (Taylor, 2016). Another prevalent issue was staffing and the level of care of each nursing assignment given. One nurse had five patients, a schizoaffective non-medicated patient, 1-day post op open reduction internal fixation of the left hip, surgical prep for a patient that had a foreign object stuck in his arm with severe cellulitis-history of intravenous drug use, suicide attempt with a sitter, and patient with chest pain with telemetry. This is a common theme of assignments nurses are facing on units and an example of unsafe staffing levels to the acuity of patients (Zysk, 2018).

The goal is to bring all concepts from the last two rotations and have a fully encompassing program that touches the issues, gaps, and probable factors that lead to workplace violence. Using the latest observations, I will start updating the workplace violence event information. At the end of this project, it is essential to have open-ended questions that pertain to these areas and how the learner feels the material will help them build stronger relationships with their patients, co-workers, and awareness to the issues to address on their units. Since this is an unusual clinical situation, the surveys will be given to those that participate in the event, online and in-person at the end of the project. The PowerPoint presentation will also be updated to address the updated material.

"Try being a rainbow in someone's cloud." ~Maya Angelou

Chapter 13

Success and Limitations of this Study

There are several factors when measuring the success or limitations of this evidence-based project. The success of the project has been the latest statistics that have emerged for patient on nurse violence, an increase of those that are willing to discuss reducing workplace violence, and the participant following the Nurses Against Violence Unite (NAVUnite) group page that was created solely to obtain further data. On the downside, reporting workplace violence is not at 100 percent, as nurses are afraid of retaliation from administration, which stem the belief of "nothing will get done as violence is a part of the job" (Speroni, Fitch, Dawson, Dugan, & Atherton, 2014, p. 219). The good thing is that the nurses joining the closed Facebook group are not shutting themselves down for change, rather watching and quietly participating in the conversation. The most recent American Nurses Association statistics contrast with what was reported last year, at 62 percent of nurses suffering verbal and physical abuse (American Nurses Association [ANA], 2018). In the January edition of American Nurse (2019), the numbers listed from the Occupational Safety and Health Commission, used to discuss workplace safety were obtained originally from the Bureau of Labor Statistics dated in 2014 (Occupational Safety and Health Administration [OSHA], n.d.). The American Nurses Association did not have actual workplace violence data until April 2018, until the "End Nurse Abuse" campaign. The downfall, not enough incidents are being reported. The reporting aspect is being covered in another project but where I have had the greatest issue regarding pulling data on injuries and verbal assaults.

Obtaining information has been done in several different forms. There have been anonymous surveys distributed for current knowledge, interviews with nursing professionals, credible online resources, nursing journals, and organizations. The online and in-person events that I have hosted to discuss the findings and to give further insight into violence in the workplace will have a final open-ended questions survey that will be offered online with a $25 gift card drawing (Moran, Burson, & Conrad, 2017). This way the nurses and nursing students will feel like they contributed valuable information and the possibility to win a prize. The benefit will increase the engagement of future material online and with the in-person events. Not to discount the fact that I will have to continue a raffle in order to keep interest and collect data. Many times, there have been nurses that have approached me behind the scenes to give information about their experiences and policies that they found regarding workplace violence and safety measures that are in place. If it was an option and funded by an organization, I would have used those funds to give gift cards to everyone that participated in the study. Throughout the time constructing and digging into the patient on nurse violence epidemic it has been a true eye-opener to the dynamic and magnitude of how workplace violence has become an expected component of nursing. Patient on nurse verbal and physical violence is a topic that is often expressed among unit colleagues as a problem area of nursing, but mainly in the emergency room or on mental health units. What I have found is that this concept is simply false. When working on medical-surgical and telemetry, while attending clinicals with students, emotions also run high on those units as well as patients that were in the emergency department are sent to the various hospital units. The fact that most emergency room nurses and mental healthcare workers are trained in de-escalation, the units are not, and the expectation is that the patient has stopped their behavior the moment they leave the ED. Speculation is speculation, but backed with experience, becoming an educator for nurses, I now see both sides from the education world to working the unit. My life as a floor CNA climbing the ranks to an Registered Nurse, 26 years seeing the shift of behaviors from nurses and patients has been unsettling. While taking the first DNP clinical rotation, I saw the organizational view of working with violent occurrences, and the follow through was not there for reporting violence. The whole experience hands-on with the personal digging into data and processes, I see the disconnects and how organizations have left us helpless and unsupported.

With the most recent statistics of 62% of nurses stated being verbally and physically assaulted, where reporting efforts have also reduced (American Nurses Association [ANA], 2018; The Joint Commission, 2018). The statistics were alarming when compared to an article reflecting that "3 out of 4 suffered physical, and 9 out of 10 nurses suffered verbal abuse", that was published 9 years ago (Chapman, 2010, para. 1). The recent reporting of events is incongruent to the current reporting efforts. The other unexpected outcome was the amount of nursing education that is in the nursing frameworks, which reflects very little about mental health or those addicted to substances. If a professor has a maternal/newborn background, she or he may not construct their material evenly with mental health intertwine as we take care of 100% of the patient, not the 25 hours that are suggested by the frameworks (Florida Department of Education [FLDOE], 2018). When I conducted a voluntary survey on the unit, every nurse discussed that they wanted to learn more so they could help the patient population heal. The social problem is that mental health and addiction has a large stigma attached to it that can be related to discrimination and make the patient feel ashamed (Davey, 2013). The nurse may or may not consciously acknowledge their own behavior towards the patient and may express undesirable verbal and non-verbal communication methods. These were the most unexpected and feel as if they are the most important besides preventing escalation to begin with.

Ethical implications would include knowing theses holes and deficits and do nothing about. It would be the desired outcome to formulate and education program to fill the gaps and bring awareness to the problem for those that are starting out in nursing. New nurses are our future and where we must prepare them for the future of our profession. The impact of the information will ripple throughout nursing, healthcare organizations, and the nursing community to bring about the change that we need. The end result will increase safety on healthcare units, assist in improving patient satisfaction scores, increase job satisfaction as nurses will feel prepared to work with those most vulnerable, and reduce job turnover.

Disseminating the findings for this project have been made through several different methods. The more scholarly way has been through social media live feeds of presentations conducted, to help nurses retrieve helpful information to help keep themselves and others safe. Working with colleagues was more difficult as their specialties would be in areas that are not exclusive to mental health or addiction. Breaking through the age-old stigma has been truly difficult as nurses have predetermined ideas about how mental health (Harmon, 2018). Most of the nurses mentioned how they did not feel prepared to care for the acute mentally ill individual. As this was made clear when using the nursing frameworks to construct the practical nursing curriculum to the set board of nursing standards (Florida Department of Education [FLDOE], 2018). When I reviewed the professional nurse standards, they were nearly identical despite the differences in job functions and responsibilities.

Presenting this information was an ongoing discovery to help nurses understand and receive the needed information to help them feel safer on their units. It was important to remain objective and honest while giving information from previous literature to fill in the gaps from where I was going with this project. The data obtained from the American Nurses Association was obtained through a survey to capture a general overview of how many nurses have been affected by violence in the workplace. There were a couple different ways that I would present this information. The first was in person, live in-services with new nurses and those preparing for graduation. Second, was through the Facebook live feature and would reach a larger audience across the United States (Moran, Burson, & Conrad, 2017). Another method could be utilizing a poster presentation to disseminate evidence-base practice to the facility to enhance or increase practice improvement (Forsyth, Wright, Scherb, & Gaspar, n.d.).

One of the main objectives is to make this education piece more widespread and help our fellow nurses to stay safe. Everywhere I go, there is some discussion about nurses and how they are not only unprepared through the nursing curriculum but also obtaining mental or physical injury. The one area that I have emphasized in this last portion of this project, is how the environment could be a factor leading to nurses to burn-out; and could be indirectly or directly causing the escalation. After the conclusion of gathering all necessary information, the dissemination of the material, and concluding the project will be a data analysis of those that participated in the training. The goal is for them to report if the education program was helpful in their practice and what other areas and what could be done to make the material more helpful to them.

The task of disseminating the result of this project had been underway for several months through gathering information and sharing the results of what was discovered along the way. Sharing the information has been through in person events and online forums through Facebook live which is progressing into webinars towards the end of this quarter. This venture will continue and will start to pick up venues through the popularity of webinars. Disseminating the findings is through webinars about nursing concerns and issues can help facilitate conversations for change within their own practice. The strength has been primarily the will to get the evidence-based and DNP project completed through the involvement of other nurses and research. The weakness is that I do not have an exuberant amount of data due to insufficient reporting of workplace violent episodes (Copeland & Henry, 2017; Sofield & Salmond, 2003; The Joint Commission, 2018). It was and still is difficult to attract experienced nurses as they may or may not be open to new information that relates to reporting or any changes due to beliefs of nothing being done and retaliation from the employer (Arnetz et al., 2015).

Poster projects are great ideas that could be utilized as another source for getting the information out to facilities to help nurses. Whether organizations would be open to having this discussion is a whole other speed bump to get over by having an open dialogue between staff and administration. By having this limitation, nurses will continue to be hurt as they are not prepared to care for those who have acute mental illness or have addiction issues. The one thing that I can say about my personal development into a scholar-practitioner and nurse leader is the sheer will to advocate for those hurting and left behind. In this case it is nurses, and ultimately the patients that we serve. If we are being attacked, there is something wrong with the structure of education and the nursing assignments that stems to how the organization is being ran.

Hurdling Barriers for Change

The pathway to achieving the Doctor of Nursing Practice credential, has been a "roll up the sleeves as I got this moment", literally from the very start. When given the opportunity to choose a topic in an area that I feel needed to be targeted for social change, I knew exactly where I needed the focus to be, workplace violence. The topic was fitting as it was the main theme throughout the beginning of the practicum and was let go due to the theme of the project. It also could be due to the involvement with the #EndNurseAbuse panel through the American Nurses Association which was a response to the Joint Commission's released sentinel event about physical and verbal abuse in the workplace (American Nurses Association [ANA], 2018). The experience was so traumatic as all I aimed to do was make a difference and help nurses to feel safe while helping others to feel better. I tried to get rehired in a hospital setting, even as a staff nurse for months as nobody in my geographical area would take a preceptee unless they were an employee or exchanged money for precepting.

Every way I turned to get help with clinical was a dead end, until the exhaustive internet search of doctorly prepared professionals and searching LinkedIn, messaging every DNP that I could find. As a result, I was lucky and grateful to have a psychologist take me under her wing. At first, she did think I was a bit manic due to the passion and excitement of relaying the research that I found, combined with explaining what happened with losing the clinical site. The key was to remain professional but in reality, I knew that I was onto something. A couple weeks went by, and my preceptor asked for the best articles to read so she could understand what I was talking about. She mentioned that it was a first for her so it was hard to digest patients attacking nurses. The next week, there was a difference in how she would discuss the issues that I presented, she understood to a degree of how extreme this problem is. Week by week she would peel back layers and realized that I may be completely right. I wanted a psychologist or a psychiatrist to assist me in this project if a DNP was unavailable, to not only validate observations but to guide me along concepts to help nurses cope, to mend relationships, and work with patients that may become combative.

The preparation to assume the leadership role is evident as my story did not start with this clinical rotation as working under challenging situations has been what I do best. Being in nursing for over 28 years now, the leadership role to advocate has taken on a new life through defending nurses with workplace violence and give them and other healthcare professionals a voice. Establishing interprofessional teams is where it would need to start as every discipline that works with patients' needs training, coping and release mechanisms, self-protection from injury and how to spot someone that could escalate. These teams would participate in the workplace violence workshops, to build comradery among each other with entertaining, interactive and guided activities. The way to establish leadership while evaluating a potentially violent situation is through practicing the behavior that you would like a participant to model. Acting responsible through providing care to everyone despite their diagnosis or situation is not only being ethical but exhibiting empathy on a consistent level to everyone you are around. I have grown a lot since starting the DNP program. The challenges I faced will always weigh heavily on me but know that no matter what came, I handled it as I would expect a leader should, never giving up or in on my beliefs or goals.

"Where the focus goes, energy flows," ~Tony Robbins

Chapter 14

Advanced Nursing Practice

The DNP essentials played a vital role in guiding the learning objectives and where I wanted to take this doctoral experience. After all these years of school, it feels as if the DNP role was completely meant for me, as it blends with my mission in life. Essential VIII is the role with previous knowledge that has given me the mastery in one area of nursing practice (American Association of Colleges of Nursing [AACN], 2006, p. 16). Forensic nursing has been my specialty, certified in 2011 and have been a certified legal nurse consultant since 2016. Doing the right thing, preparing nurses for legal and regulatory issues, including but not limiting to workplace violence. This DNP project is just the beginning of the design, implementing and therapeutic interventions that blends other sciences, such as psychology (AACN, 2006).

Promoting Quality Improvement

There a couple of areas that can be associated and pertinent to the DNP focus, organizational or system for quality improvements, including risk reduction and the promotion of health. Essential II is the realization that workplace violence either patient on nurse or horizontal violence in the workplace, ultimately affects the patient and nurse in some form or another. The goal is to eliminate health disparities and to promote patient safety (AACN, 2006). Determining the need, formal nursing education and further trainings would be needed to help determine the needs of the population. Adding the additional benefit of interjecting psychology concepts, can help a nurse to feel more fulfilled and competent to take care of her patients. Essential VII the key to heading off escalation is to watch societal trends and prevent issues prior to them becoming a problem for the patient, staff, and the organizations (AACN, 2006, p. 15). The one area that sticks out for this project, is the nursing frameworks. There is very little information to help nurses understand that they need to focus certain areas for the safety of the patient and nurse. With the increase of the opioid epidemic mixed with other substances, nurses are under the impression that since they do not work in the emergency department, that they will not see these patients come up their units. The same thought trap goes with patients will always go straight to mental health and will be medically cleared first in the ED, so they do not have to work with them. This is inaccurate. A patient does not leave their mental illness or addiction in a box or keep it in check for their visit but is one of the main reasons why they are in the hospital. Nurses are not properly prepared academically or trained through their employer of how to work with these individuals. As not being prepared leaves the nurse open for burn-out, post-traumatic stress disorder, poor job satisfaction, and turnover. All this leading to poor staffing and the increase of patient and nursing staff injuries. This is why I am working on an education plan to help nurses and nursing staff to work with potentially combative patients while developing coping skills and building relationship with patients and staff. Prevention and quality improvement are key to retaining happy and healthy nurses.

Improving Health Outcomes

Essential I reflected the complexity of the topic, workplace violence, principles and laws that govern the well-being of nurses, human behavior with building relationships and how we are as one with our environments (American Association of Colleges of Nursing [AACN], 2006, p. 9). Essential VI focus was how the multi-tiered environment, such as the administrative level to those that are on the front line of healthcare, to contribute to provide safe, timely, effective, efficient, equitable, and patient-centered care (AACN, 2006, p. 14). How does this translate with the DNP project? Sometimes by worrying about everything else at the administrative level, those that are facing the violent situations on the floor suffer without a proactive look at trends in society and education. As a nurse leader, I can bring together various interprofessional teams to collaborate and even assume the role if needed to run the team. Furthermore, effective therapeutic communication can assist in the creation or upgrade of standards of care, health policy, and practice models in complex healthcare delivery systems or issues that may arise (AACN, 2006). The re-establishment of nurses building relationships with each other and the professional nurse-patient relationship can bring about a positive change in the workplace and prevent increased anxiety due to patient hospitalization.

Holes in the Admission and Involuntary Committing Process

One of the goals of this project, was to identify other contributors how patients could escalate during a visit to a healthcare facility. In a recent study conducted nationwide found that 62% of nurses stated that they were either verbally or physically assaulted, with approximately one out of five nurses were physically attacked (American Nurses Association [ANA], 2018; Bolvin, 2018). The practicum site is a private addiction and mental illness stabilization facility, where my preceptor, is a family nurse practitioner that specializes in psychiatry and addiction. The goal for this practicum experience over the first three weeks is to get oriented to the facility, locate policies, and observe the flow of the patient admission process. During the past few weeks, I have noticed that the facility has an organized process that begins with information that has transferred from a processing or call center, located in another city. The patient could be a walk-in which is usually a voluntary admission or with a police officer, that means the patient is placed under a Baker Act (Department of Mental Health Law & Policy, 2014). It is essential to identify the different statuses as it could mean a few things that can affect a patient's behavior.

It was a great start with watching the upper management discuss their admissions process in real-time and have invited me to attend every time I am there for clinical, to get use to the team process from the top to the nurse caring for the patient. We are still trying to access different policies that are crucial to the flow of the practicum process to finding the gap in practice. Utilizing Essential II: Organizational and systems leadership for quality improvement and systems thinking is the most appropriate and fits the criteria for this practicum (American Association of Colleges of Nursing [AACN], 2006). The past few weeks have been helpful to get acclimated to the process and the beginning phases of how this practicum site admits their patients.

Working at the clinical site for this practicum has brought into perspective the various areas included in the admission process, and how an intervention to help patients would be ideal. Watching the admissions process at the receiving facility has been the only opportunity to view any holes of care. Visiting the call center is on the list of priorities to experience, pending facility approval since it is at another location. When the patient is approved with insurance verification, they will either have a transportation service, friend or family drop-off. At times there will be a police officer or a facility to facility arrangement from a hospital system. There may be an addiction, stated or observed emotional crisis where the patient needs services set-up and help to receive resources.

Statistical data reflects varying points of the enormous fluctuation of unemployment and homelessness in the United States from 2007 to 2009, which has had a great impact on mental health and the securement of employment (Bureau of Labor Statistics [BLS], 2012; Poremski, Woodhall-Melnik, Lemieux, & Stergiopoulos, 2016). In 2015, adults that have sought out mental illness care was approximately 65.7%, with an increase of those suffering, being seen in the emergency department (Office of Disease Prevention and Health Promotion [DPHP], 2018; Lochead, 2009). As the quarter moves on, the goal is to reduce patient escalation and increase communication. Options would include designating a person to discuss the process of admission or to find another means of securing the patient to feel informed of the process of admission. The person that is suffering from mental illness, addiction or both, need a structured plan of action so they can feel empowered and valued as a patient. The leadership at the center was onboard with creating an admission process sheet to include in the packet for patients. The admission process could be convoluted for someone that is withdrawing from substances. Having a sheet reiterating the process would be helpful to decrease confusion and misunderstandings. The next phase of the practicum will be the creation and implementation of this document.

The determination of how the set-up of the document will be, depends on the support or input of the administration along with key staff members. The recovery center has a plethora of individuals that come through that are either involuntarily or voluntarily committed for detox or that are suffering with acute mental illness. The intake nurse receives the admission criteria and accepts the patient, this is where the one on one care begins, and the clock starts for the proceeding events. The patient that is an involuntary hold for 72 hours, has the right to be seen within 12 to 24 hours from the facility medical provider for medical clearance and admission for mental health and detoxification (Florida Department of Children and Families [DCF], 2014; Department of Mental Health Law & Policy, 2014). During the process of arriving at the receiving center, the patient may be disoriented, disorganized in thought, having symptoms of withdraw, including but not limited to anxiety or delusions (Gilbert, 2009). Others that play an intricate roll within the 72-hour window include the psychiatric nurse practitioner, the case manager, interim therapist, an assigned therapist for on-going therapy, and a financial officer.

For many that are actively experiencing withdrawal, non-violent euphoria, delusions, or anxiety, knowing the steps of their care is an integral part of their recovery. One of the main goals for this practicum project was to simplify the process and have something for the patient to refer back to when they arrive. With the guidance of my preceptor and the existing information from the welcome packets, the simplified version of the process sheet was created. Simple, and to the point. The proposal for the admission process outline is for placement in the admission welcome packets and on the walls of the common areas. To create this change, there are a few more levels in corporate that need to approve of this additional support of the current procedures. In the meantime, nurses are using the document when patients forget the next step in their care.

Process of Admission

Day One

Arriving to the facility, you can expect:

1. Belongings checked in.
2. Meet with the intake nurse for the initial assessments.

Within 24 hours you will also meet:

1. MD or Nurse Practitioner for a health evaluation.
2. Therapy will go over a background, events and factors that brought you here with us.

Day Two

Within 48 to 72 hours the Psychiatrist or Psychiatric Nurse Practitioner will

- Mental health history
- Discuss possible treatment options

Day Three

Medical Follow-up with a Medical Doctor or Family Nurse Practitioner:

- Detoxing – Daily for withdrawal symptoms
- Partial Hospitalization Program (PHP) & Residential – 1 x week
- Intensive Outpatient – 1 x month

Required to attend group therapy:

- Detoxing - *Encouraged to attend*
- Partial Hospitalization Program (PHP)
- Residential
- Intensive Outpatient (IOP)

By the completion of the 72 hours you will have met:

1. Case Manager
2. Therapist
3. Financial Officer

Credential prepared by: Sandra Risoldi MSN Ed., RN, CLNC

Chapter 15

Creating a Workplace Violence Policy

These topics strike a chord, and practicum focus hits every point of this discussion. There are many issues regarding workplace violence and the components that tag along which are ethical issues, reporting violent situations, communication deficiencies, including but not limited to building relationships with peers and patients. When there is workplace violence, we can automatically point the cause is from lateral or horizontal violence, where it can be defined as "verbal threats, intimidation, or coercion" from another staff member (Taylor, 2016, p. 5). Workplace violence policies are generally zero tolerance, but effective implementation has failed or not enforced (Paterson, Miller, Bowie, & Ledbetter, 2008). The facility where I am attending practicum is a substance recovery center and does not have a workplace violence policy in place. The only rule that stands out in the employee handbook is to follow the chain of command in case of a disagreement among staff. According to essential V, "DNP graduates are prepared to design, influence, and implement healthcare policies" (American Association of Colleges of Nursing [AACN], 2006, p. 13). In this case, there is no policy for workplace violence and incivility among peers which can directly affect the safety of patients and staff.

The DNP leader can change the face of nursing. This can be achieved by creating a plan, put it into action by advocating for the change of policy and social injustices (AACN, 2006). We have nurses suffering burn-out, post-traumatic stress disorder, and many leaving nursing or turning over into other positions to escape the lack of support and resources that nurses should have to care for patients (Ashton, Morris, & Smith, 2017; Mealer, Burnham, Goode, Rothbaum, & Moss, 2009). The most recent survey from the American Nurses Association (2018) states that 62% of nurses reported having been physically and verbally abused. The statistics are not even accurate and severely underreported (Paterson et al., 2008). If all nurses reported workplace violence, we would see a massive shift in how organizations function and hopefully change would be enacted in legislation. As for the facility where I am precepting, it would be essential to take action one step at a time and help them formulate a workplace violence policy.

1) Currently the facility where I attend clinical, there is a verbal understanding about chain of command and what to do if a patient starts to escalate. The procedure in place is the nurse calls a code overhead and someone designated from the other floors comes to assist in de-escalation. The facility does not have a workplace violence policy of any kind and the training that was in place is no longer being provided, due to the employee's separation. When the nurse goes to report the problem, there is no reporting structure to follow. If there is a serious enough injury, the nurse will be sent to the emergency department for a drug test and assessment of injuries. This would be the only time there will be a report filled out to worker's compensation for the injury. As far as barriers, it would revolve around educating the staff and ensuring there are policies in place to protect the staff member, the patient, and facility against liability. On the flip side, another facility that I was attending had a reporting system that pointed to a miscellaneous file where the focus was on near misses and medical mishaps. There were policies in place and the nurses reported in anonymous surveys that they do not feel anything happens when they do report, which is echoed throughout nursing literature (American Nurses Association [ANA], 2018; Ashton, Morris, & Smith, 2017; Bolvin, 2018; Mealer, Burnham, Goode, Rothbaum, & Moss, 2009; Paterson, Miller, Bowie,

& Ledbetter, 2008; Speroni, Fitch, Dawson, Dugan, & Atherton, 2014; The Joint Commission, 2018; Trinkoff et al., n.d.).

2) Throughout this DNP program, I picked a hot topic due to the desire to change the direction of nursing by bringing it in the future. My comfort is high when finding holes in organizational structure and advocating for those it affects. Thinking back to when I started out in nursing, I always wanted to work for the Joint Commission. Working agency as a LPN, the facilities would have them follow me, as their staff was not proficient for Joint Commission to observe and what was told to me after when getting hours signed. As for a personal role after finishing the DNP program is well defined and the path for me is revealing itself a new layer everyday. Right now, I am working on two books, in the Fall I may take the Psychiatric Mental Health Nurse Practitioner post-master's certificate to solidify my role as a well-rounded forensic nurse. I will be starting educational webinars about workplace violence and nursing issues, attending speaking engagements about the psychology behind what nurses are going through, and advocate for nurses at a legislative level, while aiming to speak in the Senate. To stay up to date with research, I belong to The American Psychological Association, Sigma Theta Tau Honor Society – Phi Nu Chapter, National Society of Leadership and Success, and the Golden Key International Honour Society.

Informing Health Care Policy

The main goal has been to analyze and define what is happening throughout healthcare system when it came to the nursing indicators and every tie into why violence in nursing has not been exposed to how we are going to fix it. When putting together a rough estimate of costs of nursing turnover, it was estimated that when a nurse leaves the system, it costs approximately

$200,000 to advertise, interview, hire, and train the new employee. If there is about 20 nurses that leave per year, the company spent a modest $4,000,000 instead of finding out why and retain the nurses, ultimately saving the company. What I have learned and good at, is the art of picking down a process and find out how it can work better and more efficiently. Between nurse and patient injuries that occur due to either verbal or physical injuries, time off either voluntary or involuntary through workers compensation only eats up resources and costing the company more money. Through introducing the webinars that I am going to start working on, book, possibly get assistance with publishing in scholarly articles, it is my passion to talk about all issues in nursing, help to make it safe, and be a support system for nurses that feel helpless in their roles.

"Respect starts with yourself." ~Napoleon Hill

Chapter 16

The Last Rotation Countdown

The ongoing efforts of this project will not be permanently concluded, as I am planning on creating a teaching plan from this project. The goal is to help nurses learn coping mechanisms, bring awareness and insight to the problem while preventing further mental or physical injuries. The post-graduation plan is to get accepted in the Psychiatric Mental Health Nurse Practitioner program, open a health and recovery facility, possibly just sober living that caters to healthcare and first responders. The goal is to help the patient whether addicted or suffering from mental illness, and to get back on their feet with medication stabilization and rehabilitation, sign a contract of continuing services in a technical program and help them to get back on their feet permanently. During the transition, the individual will also have room and board in a recovery house while attending school. In addition to opening a facility, I am starting to speak in schools, and would like to extend the opportunity to healthcare facilities, conferences, and hold online webinars or workshops for learners to gain more knowledge. We are working on a certification program and eventually offer continuing education credits.

Over the last two years, I have been uncovering various holes within the reporting system, observing behaviors of peers, and the pattern of interactions between patients, their families, and staff. While working with the preceptor who has her psychology degree, it has taken me from seeing one side of the issue, as patients being the only causation of nursing injuries. When it has been a variety of factors to cause the escalation of behavior in patients and nurses. Even though I saw what was going on way before the first meeting with my psychology preceptor, she guided me to make sound decisions of the direction of this project. It has been a very long road to convey these issues without judgment from peers, employers, preceptors and even some faculty as it is hard to believe that nurses could hold some of the burden of liability in the creation of the escalation. It is obvious that this project about nursing violence has not been popular with organizations as they could have been determined as a threat, which has never been my intention. The intention is to prepare and release a series of the project broken down on YouTube in hopes that it will bring awareness to the problems to the issues that nurses face. Some of the issues that I had faced throughout this program have been traumatic yet persevered due to my moral compass and drive to help nurses to not only be safe but love their jobs without retaliation.

It was told to me that I was let go from the hospital clinical rotation due to the involvement with the American Nurses Association End Nurse Abuse panel, the latest Sentinel Event from The Joint Commission, compounded with finding holes in the hospital reporting system. The mentioned holes in the reporting system were found before the Joint Commission (2018) number 59 on verbal and physical violence and how incidences were underreported. Many nurses are getting injured due to the frameworks that limit mental health and addiction to approximately 25 hours and not regarded as a crucial role in patient care, only as a specialization. The standard should be across the board for mental health to be integrated into all board of nursing frameworks (Florida Department of Education [FLDOE], 2018). Was this okay to accept and look away as just another completed project? No. After being let go from the hospital rotation, with much sadness, the girls and I relocated to Orlando. It worked itself out and was able to get experienced a DNP along with the psychologist (located in Tampa) preceptor. As a result, I was able to do a staff education project versus a systematic literature review, which was not what I wanted to achieve for the DNP project. It is my passion to continue to reach out to students, experienced nurses, nurses' aides, patient care technicians, administrators, and anyone that will listen, about decreasing violence in the workplace, both laterally and from patients. Building relationships across the lines and hopes that I can mend mental health and medical together, even more, to provide nurses and patients with a better environment for healing.

After the conclusion of the DNP, one goal is to continue learning and receive a Psychiatric Mental Health Nurse Practitioner post-master's certification, then open a facility focusing on health and recovery. The goal is to not call it a mental health or addiction facility, due to the enormous amount of stigma associated with addiction and mental illness, it is detrimental to steer away from labeling words with negative undertones. The idea behind this concept is when the person is discharged to facility-type home or otherwise called a half-way house, they will receive free room and board while enrolled in a technical college or trade program. When they graduate, they will give back by volunteering to help those who need a role-model and sponsor. The facility will also be nurse ran and centered, along with our technicians and nurses' aides, ensuring that all staff is protected and valued. They will have shared governance and assist with policy upgrades and protections. The more immediate goal is to continue the classes on speaking and start educational webinars which are underway.

Ultimately, building a solid following and change the culture of nursing from "violence is a part of the job" to educate, empower and eliminate violence in the workplace. To engage more in the professional organizations that I am a current member of the National Society of Leadership and Success, Golden Key International Honour Society, Sigma Theta Tau Honor Society of Nursing – Phi Nu Chapter, the Honor Society and the American Psychological Association. It is a goal to also play an active role to secure speaking engagements and join forces to speak in the Senate about workplace violence as well as the board of nursing to increase the curriculum frameworks for mental health and addiction education.

The focus of this rotation is to continue implementing the educational program, evaluate the effectiveness of the learned material from the stakeholders, and disseminate the information as a final project for this practicum. During the re-evaluation phase of the last practicum, I met with my preceptor to discuss where we left off and where I see the remainder of the project going for this final phase. We discussed the different areas previously covered, including the relationship between patients and nurses, verbal and non-verbal communication techniques to decrease patient on nurse violence, and coping mechanisms. This rotation will continue to focus on the nurse-patient relationship. The goal is to analyze how external stimuli and an increased patient workload can affect morale, the strain on nurses to perform for the organization, which can directly or indirectly result in verbal and physical abuse from patients (Fasanya & Dada, 2015). The essentials were adjusted to precisely align the objectives throughout the project.

It is important to continue researching and recalling previous information to incorporate into this final rotation. The goal was to find environmental factors that could bring about negative behavior in both nurse and patient. A few areas right away observed was the lighting, call bells, telemetry monitors, intravenous medication pumps, and the noise of conversations being held at the nurse's station. While standing for a few minutes observing the workflow, you can hear gossip and snarky comments about the prior shift. There was another episode where a nurse made comments of the night shift having it "easy as they did not have all of the responsibilities they did on days." The discussions on the unit between staff were minimal, but there were also nonverbal eye-rolling and dirty looks when asked to help another nurse out in a crunch situation (Taylor, 2016). Another prevalent issue was staffing and the level of care of each nursing assignment given. One nurse had five patients, a schizoaffective non-medicated patient, 1-day post op open reduction internal fixation of the left hip, surgical prep for a patient that had a foreign object stuck in his arm with severe cellulitis-history of intravenous drug use, suicide attempt with a sitter, and patient with chest pain with telemetry. This is a common theme of assignments nurses are facing on units and an example of unsafe staffing levels to the acuity of patients (Zysk, 2018).

The start of this practicum rotation was more comfortable, with a better understanding of the admissions process, it was time to find other areas that have not been addressed. When arriving, my preceptor and I went over this quarter's rotation to ensure this writer did not previously cover the objectives. The idea is to introduce new concepts of prevention and enhance current policy to help reduce or eliminate patient on nurse violence. The goal over the next few weeks is to observe the workflow among therapists, nurses, doctors, and nurse practitioners while reviewing the reporting mechanisms that are currently in place. During the observation period, some additional activities included locating the current policy on workplace violence. The policy is still being located and may create one to help them along if they do not have one in place.

When determining the extent of the violence that nurses experience, prior data needed to be obtained if the facility had not been reporting all incidents. An overview of national or local statistics would be necessary to see the magnitude of violent occurrences. In 2014, nurses ranging from "26 to 64 years" of age, with a significant amount of experience, reported approximately "76 percent experienced violence, 54 percent verbal and 30 percent physical attacks" (Speroni, Fitch, Dawson, Dugan, & Atherton, 2014, p. 218). A few years later, the American Nurses Association (2018) conducted a survey revealing that 62 percent of nurses stated that they have both verbally and physically abused which numbers were much higher, yet vastly underreported (The Joint Commission, 2018). While reviewing the National Database of Nursing Quality Indicators, several areas seemed to connect and feed into one significant problem, job satisfaction, and turnover as a possible result from psychiatric, physical assaults (Montalvo, 2007). The next few weeks will focus on actual reporting, shift reports, where does the report go when collected, and what is the process of action to prevent or correct future occurrences.

A continuation of observation of the units, how nurses are reporting events and the flow of interaction between the nurse, patient and other interdisciplinary members that assist with daily care. There have been many times that I have seen patients become upset about situations or not feeling well and lash out at staff. The episode that I witnessed involved two patients that were arguing about something relating to food, lunging toward each other and looked as if they were going to fight. Watching the nurses getting upset over feeling like they have lost control of the situation, the lack of security poses a higher risk for injury to both the patients and staff that is there to diffuse the situation (Angland, Dowling, & Casey, 2013). Minor to major mental health morbidities have been associated with high-stress environments which can cause anger, anxiety, depressed mood, mental fatigue, burn-out, and adjustment disorders (Trinkoff et al., n.d.).

Another component to why violence has increased on healthcare units is also due to administrators that consider violence as a part of the job, increasing the fear of retaliation that if the nurse reports the issue, that the nurse is incompetent to perform (Speroni, Fitch, Dawson, Dugan, & Atherton, 2014; Trinkoff et al., n.d.). To take the theory a step farther, the demonization of the nurse that reported, results in the nurse learning to become helpless and does not try to change the situation (Ashton, Morris, & Smith, 2017). The good thing is that the facility is about to change leadership soon to also ensure the nursing staff feels protected and the delivery of quality care is present. As a result of the growing escalation in the facility, I was asked to create a generic workplace violence policy and reporting structure to help all of the healthcare workers know the correct reporting procedures.

Reflecting on the time completed throughout the last two quarters, this has been a wonderful yet very stressful experience. So, the saying goes, a little pain only helps on get to the next level both personally and professionally. During my time with these rotations, I have witnessed and contributed to bringing awareness and safety education to nursing staff, while assisting in the creation of a workplace violence policy. What happens after this week…the final week? I still have some project fine tuning to complete, a bit upset about it, but again, the pain is needed to grow into a quality DNP practitioner. Coming from an extremely humble background, being homeless, abused as a child, left behind at 16 years old, fending for myself well before then, and achieving a GED not even finishing the 9th grade, I can honestly say this is my time. Bold goals for Nurses Against Violence Unite, Inc., as it is detrimental to our profession by navigating change in nursing by giving unwavering support and advocate for those that are afraid to speak on their own due to retaliation from their employers or simply not ready. So many things have happened with Nurses Against Violence Unite, Inc. and feel as if this was a calling to serve, connect, and be the support system for the front lines of healthcare.

Conclusion

When deciding to work on violence and reporting issues in nursing, it was something I shook my head, looked at my co-worker saying, this is going to either make a lot of people mad at first but reveal that it is the total system failure which has affected the safety and morale of nursing. It has not helped matters with surveys for patient satisfaction to weigh in on service of the nursing staff. The system is broken. After deciding on the topic for the DNP project, it was so hard to narrow it down and attempted to make it as focused as possible, on one concept, preventing patient on nurse abuse through education, in verbatim and copywritten form, I have included it in this publication for review. Simultaneously working on Nurses Against Violence Unite, Inc.™ to bring awareness, educate, empower and eliminate violence in nursing, it has grown exponentially to a global effort and increasing in size by the day. We held our first rally in Washington, DC on August 2, 2019. We have been featured on the hit TV series "The

Doctors", The KC Ingram Show https://vimeo.com/351037155, assisted with stories for ABC news affiliate WHAS11 with Paula Vasan, FOX news affiliate Fox channel 4 Kansas City Missouri Lisa McCormick "State director says violence against nurses is an epidemic in Missouri and nationwide," Nurse.com, and The Eye on Health, now called The Medical Beat, FM Radio 97.1 Missouri with Dr. Steve Harvey. In August 2020, I was chosen from thousands of applicants, by the prestigious organization American Psychological Association (APA) to speak about the violence that is occurring with frontline healthcare workers. The topic of workplace violence is not the vision of what we would think of when it comes to nursing care, definitely not a popular topic but one that is completely necessary in recent times. We are losing nurses to burn-out, PTSD from traumatic events, physical injuries, and the lack of resources that make nurses feel that no matter what they do, nothing will ever get better, trapping them into learned helplessness. What is learned helplessness? It is when no matter how hard we try to help and do what is right for our patients or fix a situation that is detrimental for safe patient care or even report incidents, we are either retaliated against for reporting the incident or treated terribly by upper management that we are not doing a good enough job and retaliated against to the point of leaving the job, continuing to excel in our roles to get out of bedside care or some leave nursing altogether. Our time is now, it is time to change the culture of nursing and unite. If you have a friend or family member that is a nurse, nursing staff or in school to become a nurse, please have them come visit our group. Nurses Against Violence Unite, Inc.™ leads the way in providing a safe space for frontline healthcare workers to report their experiences anonymously, talk about issues that they are facing and feel like they are a part of a big family, working together to eliminate violence in the workplace.

"Create a vision and never let the environment, other people's beliefs, or the limits of what has been done in the past shape your decisions." ~Tony Robbins

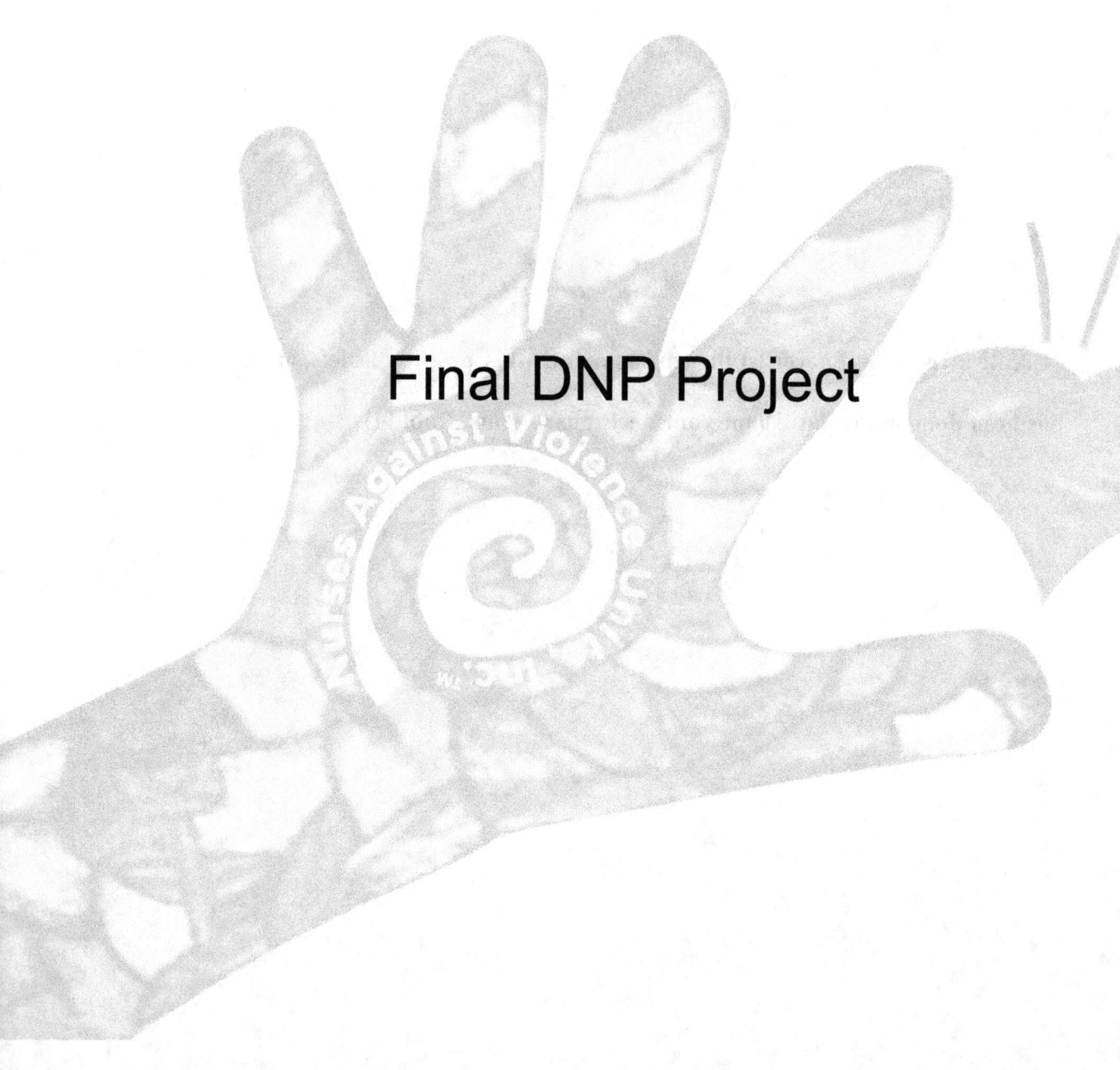
Final DNP Project

Walden University

College of Health Sciences

This is to certify that the doctoral study by

Sandra Risoldi

has been found to be complete and satisfactory in all respects, and that any and all revisions required by the review committee have been made.

Review Committee

Dr. Cassandra Taylor, Committee Chairperson, Nursing Faculty
Dr. Mary Martin, Committee Member, Nursing Faculty
Dr. Jonas Nguh, University Reviewer, Nursing Faculty

Chief Academic Officer Eric Riedel, Ph.D.

Walden University

2019

Abstract

Preventing Patient on Nurse Violence Through Education

by

Sandra L. Risoldi

MSN Ed., Walden University, 2017

BSN, South University, 2014

Project Submitted in Partial Fulfillment of the
Requirements for the Degree of

Doctor of Nursing Practice

Walden University

June 2019

Abstract

Many nurses are physically and verbally abused by the patients under their care, with those providing care to patients dealing with mental illness or addition being at particular risk. Leadership of the project site, an urban mental health treatment center, identified a need to provide additional education to improve their nursing staff's ability to work with combative patients and prevent escalation of violent behaviors. Albert Bandura's social cognitive theory and adaptation to the environment guided the development of this project to answer the question if an education program for nurses working with potentially combative patients will increase their knowledge of strategies to prevent escalation of violent behavior. The education program was developed using results from an extensive literature review and input from a team of local subject experts, who provided evaluation regarding their satisfaction with the planning process through the completion of an anonymous, 10 questions, Likert-type survey. All team members scored each question with a (5) strongly agree or (4) agree. Project deliverables handed over to the facility included the developed education program, an associated handout, a plan for later implementation, and plans for outcome evaluation through evaluation of learning. This project has the potential to achieve positive social change through less violent encounters between nurses and patients, contributing to an increased culture of safety.

Preventing Patient on Nurse Violence Through Education

by

Sandra L. Risoldi

MSN Ed., Walden University, 2017

BSN, South University, 2014

Project Submitted in Partial Fulfillment of the
Requirements for the Degree of

Doctor of Nursing Practice

Walden University

June 2019

Table of Contents

Section 1: Nature of the Project 1

    Introduction 1

    Problem Statement 2

    Purpose 3

    Nature of the Doctoral Project 3

    Significance 4

    Summary 4

Section 2: Background and Context 6

    Introduction 6

    Concepts, Models, and Theories 6

    Relevance to Nursing Practice 7

    Local Background and Context 13

    Role of the Doctor of Nursing Practice Student 14

    Role of the Project Team 15

    Summary 15

Section 3: Collection and Analysis of Evidence 17

    Introduction 17

    Practice-Focus Question 18

    Sources of Evidence 18

    Program Development 19

    Analysis and Synthesis 20

Summary 20

Section 4: Findings and Recommendations 22

    Introduction 22

    Findings and Implications 23

    Recommendations 27

    Contributions of the Doctoral Project Team 28

    Strengths and Limitations of the Project 29

Section 5: Dissemination Plan 30

    Dissemination Plan 30

    Analysis of Self 30

    Summary 31

References 33

Appendix A: Evaluation Questionnaire for Team of Experts 41

Appendix B: Behavior Prevention Educational Program 42

Appendix C: Education Handout 49

Appendix D: Educational Program Comprehension Questionnaire 50

Section 1: Nature of the Project

Introduction

Verbal and physical violence against nurses is growing at an epidemic rate. The American Nurses Association (ANA, 2018) #EndNurseAbuse survey revealed out of 14,000 nurses who responded, 62% stated they had suffered both physical and verbal abuse from patients. The most recent report reflects that interactions with patients caused 80% of nurse injuries, and 17,000 violence-related injuries occurred in a combination of hospital and long-term care facilities (Esposito, 2017, Occupational Safety and Health Administration [OSHA], 2015). Among hospital departments, emergency departments contain multiple risk factors for patient-on-nurse violence. Over the last 10 years in the United States, the number of patients visiting the emergency department has grown from 90.3 million to 119.2 million, with psychiatric visits increasing to 2.89 million per year (Florida Council for Community Mental Health, 2011). Among those admitted to the emergency department, there has been an increase number of patients with acute mental illness and substance abuse; who are brought in by law enforcement officers for medical clearance, admission, and observation (Gacki-Smith et al., 2009).

While the emergency department staff often receives training for de-escalation of potentially violent patients, few nurses on the general and intensive hospital units have been formally trained with an escalation behavior management program. When a patient is admitted to an observation bed, it could be on a medical-surgical, orthopedics, telemetry, or a stand-alone observation unit where the nurse may or may not have had specific escalation behavior management training. The project site is a specialty unit, providing care during recovery from acute mental illness, drugs and alcohol. Staff in this setting have a greater understanding of working with this population but felt the need to improve their knowledge with a focus on prevention of violent behavior escalation. The purpose of this project was to develop an education program for nursing staff regarding strategies to prevent escalation of violent behavior in combative patients. The projected positive social change of this doctoral project is to prevent behavior escalation, thereby reducing patient-on-nurse violence and subsequent physical and mental injury.

Problem Statement

The ANA (2018) #EndNurseAbuse survey revealed that out of 14,000 nurses who responded, 62% stated they had suffered both physical and verbal abuse from patients. Violence is affecting nurses in various ways. Nurses may suffer from burn-out or posttraumatic stress disorder, which leads to the reduction of productivity, an increase in call-offs, and high turnover rates (Gates, Gillespie, & Succop, 2011). The morale of the nursing population is being negatively affected by the growing number of violent episodes against nurses.

The local problem is that the selected urban hospital's leadership has recognized the need to provide additional education for staff to improve their nursing staff's ability to work with combative patients and prevent escalation. Currently, there is no formal continuing education in place at this facility. Pre-licensure education for the practical and professional nursing program, provide approximately 25 hours of mental illness and addiction training. The combination of minimal formal nursing education requirements and little to no continuing education in the healthcare setting means that experienced nurses and new graduates are not prepared to work with behavior escalation (Zhao et al., 2015).

Purpose

The purpose of this project was to develop an education program for nursing staff regarding strategies to prevent escalation of violent behavior in combative patients. The gap in practice is that nurses are not prepared to prevent violence escalation, due to the lack of knowledge of how to work with combative patients. Provision of continuing education may address this practice gap by providing nurses with information on strategies to prevent escalation. The guiding question for this project was: Will an education program for nurses working with potentially combative patients increase their knowledge of strategies to prevent escalation of violent behavior?

Nature of the Doctoral Project

In order to develop a staff education program for staff nurses, it was essential to conduct a literature search for several key terms referencing workplace violence while utilizing the team of local experts. Incorporating evidence from the literature, along with valuable input from the team, I developed an education program tailored to the organization's need. The interdisciplinary team consisted of a physician, a family nurse practitioner (FNP), and a staff nurse, all experts within their profession. The purpose of this project was to develop an education program for nursing staff regarding strategies to prevent escalation of violent behavior in combative patients. The gap in practice is that nurses are not prepared to prevent violence escalation, due to the lack of knowledge of how to work with combative patients.

Significance

The stakeholders identified are the nurse managers, staff nurses, therapists, ancillary staff, and patients. Staff nurses, ancillary staff and therapists would be affected since they work directly with the patient population and at a higher risk for being injured. When working with potentially combative patients, education is key to reducing injury by increasing skills to manage the risk. Other stakeholders are the patients on the healthcare unit, who are witness to escalation during the day or at night, are at a higher risk for sleep disturbance, affecting the patient's healing process (Stiver et al., 2017). Nursing managers and administrators are stakeholders, since this education could assist in the creation and maintenance of a culture of safety.

The potential impact on nursing practice will be a decrease in violent acts against nurses, an increase in morale, improved working conditions, increased self-efficacy, and decreasing turnover rates. This project has transferability to any workplace where nurses care for patients who are at risk for violent behaviors, which essentially is any area where nurses work. This project has the potential to influence positive social change by decreasing violence in health care environments and protecting both nurses and their patients.

Summary

The ANA (2018) #EndNurseAbuse survey revealed out of 14,000 nurses who responded, 62% stated they had suffered both physical and verbal abuse from patients. The gap in practice is that nurses are not prepared to prevent violence escalation, due to the lack of knowledge of how to work with combative patients. The purpose of this project was to develop an education program for nursing staff regarding strategies to prevent escalation of violent behavior in combative patients. The guiding question for this project was: Will an education program for nurses working with potentially combative patients increase their knowledge of strategies to prevent escalation of violent behavior? The goal is to prevent escalation of violent encounters with combative patients.

Section 2: Background and Context

Introduction

The ANA (2018) #EndNurseAbuse survey revealed out of 14,000 nurses who responded, 62% stated they had suffered both physical and/or verbal abuse from patients. The purpose of this project was to develop an education program for nursing staff regarding strategies to prevent escalation of violent behavior in combative patients. The guiding question for this project was: Will an education program for nurses working with potentially combative patients increase their knowledge of strategies to prevent escalation of violent behavior? The goal is to prevent escalation of violent encounters with combative patients. Utilizing established concepts such as the social cognitive theory, along with the subcomponent's resilience and adaptation, the staff education program was created for the facility by the interprofessional team of experts.

Concepts, Models, and Theories

Albert Bandura was the sole creator of the social cognitive theory, which evolved originally from the social learning theory in the 1960s and separated in 1986 where the learning involves the return of the same behavior from the person within the environment (LaMorte, 2018). The social cognitive theory is best explained when personal experiences, life events, behavioral patterns, mixed with environmental factors interact with another, influencing each other (Bandura, 2001). Belief systems can play a role in how the patient or nurse is perceived during care by anticipating behavior that could arise during a hospital stay (Bandura, 1989). Through social cognitive therapy, it is suggested that the behavior exhibited from nurses and patients may model one's behavior or actions (Sidhu & Park, 2018). Ultimately resulting in the patient perception of the nurse's reactions as a reason to escalate or become combative.

The use of the adaptation theory, a component of the social cognitive theory, enables the nurse to take control of their actions and thoughts, through finding the meaning behind the violent event (Benight & Bandura, 2003; Chapman, Styles, Perry, & Combs, 2010). When a nurse experiences a traumatic event, they start to adapt to the behavior by searching for another meaning, attempting to understand the situation and adjust their behavior to better themselves (Taylor, 1983). If the nurse does not recognize the need for an outlet to cope with the on-going stressful events of the healthcare environment, it can lead to compassion fatigue, burn-out, and post-traumatic stress disorder, reducing the ability to adapt (Schmidt & Haglund, 2017). The connection between the adaptation theory and this education program, is the nurse will adapt to the environment by remaining free from verbal and physical abuse and gain knowledge to effectively work with combative patients.

Relevance to Nursing Practice

Recent statistics revealed that a large number of nurse respondents have suffered and reported verbal and physical abuse, resulting in the need for training and subsequent educational training opportunities (ANA, 2018; Bolvin, 2018; Florida Department of Education [FLDOE], 2018). Studies have revealed a relationship between substance abuse and patient aggression in the healthcare setting (American College of Emergency Physicians [ACEP], 2009; Kleissl-Muir, Raymond, & Rahman, 2018). The nursing school curriculum in Florida, for both practical and professional nurse programs, have minimal requirements for addressing mental health and substance abuse. One full section addresses communication and interprofessional skills, and three subheadings address care planning for a psychiatric patient, defense mechanisms, and adverse effects of substance abuse (FLDOE, 2018). When creating a course curriculum, the nursing instructor is given the autonomy to address the depth and amount of education on a determined subject, within the approved guidelines. The amount of education for each section is not standardized; as a result, if the instructor that creates the course curriculum is not proficient in the area, then the area may not have extensive detail. Insufficient mental health and substance abuse training in both the practical and professional nursing curriculum may contribute to the epidemic of patient violence against nurses (FLDOE, 2018).

The recent statistical data released from the ANA (2018) #EndNurseAbuse survey revealed out of 14,000 nurses who responded, 62% stated they had suffered both physical and verbal abuse from patients. Bolvin (2018) released further statistics that one in five nurses reported a physical assault, where 42 percent made a written report, and nearly half of those who did report were not satisfied with the outcome of the incident. The incidence of underreporting workplace violence can be contributed to the beliefs of nurses that nothing will get done, violence is a part of the job, nobody was hurt, and the violence may be unintentional due to the patient's condition (Sofield & Salmond, 2003; Chojnacka, 2005; Snyder, Chen, & Vacha-Haase, 2007; Gates et al., 2011; Sato, Wakabayashi, Kiyoshi-Teo, & Fukahori, 2012; Arnetz et al., 2015; Hogarth, Beattie, & Morphet, 2015; Copeland & Henry, 2017; The Joint Commission, 2018; American

Nurses Association [ANA], 2018; Bolvin, 2018). From an administrative standpoint, reported data are the only way that an issue can be identified (The Joint Commission, 2018). Gates (2011) has also further suggested that organizations do not favor reporting as it may directly affect the patient satisfaction scores. If no statistical data can be retrieved in the system, then there will be no evidence of a problem.

A recent study was conducted on the effects of patient-inflicted violence towards nurses, resulting in burnout and nursing turnover (Laeeque, Bilal, Babar, Khan, & Rahman, 2017). The research was conducted between four hospitals, 350 questionnaires were sent to the human resources department where they were distributed among the participants and the ability to remain anonymous over the study's three-month period (Laeeque et al., 2017). The result of the research concluded that patient on nurse violence increased occupational stress, leading to burn-out, directly and indirectly resulting in staff turnover (Laeeque et al., 2017). Recommendations from the research suggested the benefit of building social groups for nurses to vent their concerns, giving advice, blogging, and attending online communities are one way to help nurses cope with the stressors they face on healthcare units (Laeeque et al., 2017).

The Agency for Healthcare Research and Quality (AHRQ) performed a systematic literature review of strategies geared towards the de-escalation of aggressive behavior that could potentially eliminate the need for seclusion or restraints through prevention measures (2016). The AHRQ (2016) suggested several avenues in the study to help reduce or enhance the milieu on the unit, including; the increase of staffing ratios, decrease the noise or chaotic environments, and utilize risk assessments on patients to prevent triggers and prevent behavior escalation. In addition to the unit modification suggestions, the use of cognitive behavior techniques, non-verbal support, and treatment of the underlying psychiatric or medical condition, could play a major part in preventing escalation (AHRQ, 2016). The presented study in the systematic literature review consisted of data captured from both men and women psychiatric patients from 38 to 40 years of age, with any ethnic background (AHRQ, 2016). The conclusive results pointed to the use of a risk assessment tool as the most effective with the reduction of seclusion and restraints in the acute care hospital. It was shown that increasing staff training and interpersonal communication skills fostered the relationship between patient and nurse, ultimately reducing the need for de-escalation procedures and prevented occurrences (AHRQ, 2016).

The next article reviewed demonstrated that staff education training decreased the use of seclusion and restraints throughout 12 months. The goals of the training program were to 1) increase awareness of what could increase behavior; 2) promote knowledge and use less restrictive measures to reduce behavior; 3) increase knowledge and training to staff to know how to react to the behavior. The training also included the hands-on simulation of being in a 5-point restraining system to provide a real example of how it must feel for the patient, also reminding learners of patient rights to reduce the more aggressive approach. By using a preventative approach with verbal interventions, self-defense training, and role-play, the annual rate of restraint use went down an overall 13.8 percent and staff injuries reduced by 18.8 percent in two-years (Forster, Cavness, & Phelps, 1999).

Another article focused on the surveillance of three hospitals and fourteen acute mental health wards, with a total of 5,384 admissions, over a three-year time frame (Bowers et al., 2006). Psychiatric staff reported feelings of guilt, self-blame, anger, anxiety, post-traumatic stress disorder, and feelings of shame following an increase of attacks from patients. The organization developed a prevention program that aimed to manage violence and aggression through education regarding how to break away from a patient attack or hold, legalities of restraining individuals, and how to manually restrain until treatment was rendered. The training program originated as a five-day course within the prison system and was modified to meet the needs of the healthcare providers working with those that have addiction and acute mental illness (Bowers et al., 2006).

The use of the six core strategies, formulated by the National Association of State Mental Health Program Directors, was beneficial in the creation of this education project (National Association of State Mental Health Program Directors [NASMHPD], 2006). Strategy steps within this article are used to reduce the need for restraints and seclusion through cooperation of patients and the prevention of behavior escalation. The areas of focus are on organizational leadership, data collection of possible deficiencies, education development, restraint/seclusion prevention tools, consumer involvement in care, and debriefing techniques (NASMHPD, 2006). One proponent that is echoed throughout this article, would be the education strategies, and how it is necessary to gather input from an interdisciplinary team and the need for a proactive leadership. Data were gathered from reported incidents advancement of the education piece through modifications and updates. The involvement of the senior level staff would prove beneficial and create a culture of reporting and promotion of safety (NASMHPD, 2006). To tie in the benefits and disadvantages of using the six core strategies, it is necessary to evaluate the effectiveness of the steps, to ensure all possible interventions were utilized during the debriefing which is held approximately 24 to 48 hours concluding the seclusion and restraint event (NASMHPD, 2006).

The Substance Abuse and Mental Health Services Administration aims to reduce the number of restraints and seclusion. Aligning insights with NASMHPD, SAMHSA has a comprehensive training program that includes the six core strategies and links inadequate staffing as a contributor to injuries, abuses, and even deaths as the result of using seclusion and restraints (Substance Abuse and Mental Health Services Administrations [SAMHSA], 2005). Through using restraints and seclusion techniques, staff could suffer secondary traumatization, which can mimic post-traumatic stress disorder when either being involved in an episode or witnessing the traumatic event (SAMHSA, 2005). Staff trained to decrease the use of restraints and seclusion did not expect the techniques to be effective, but combative behavior and injuries decreased after the training (O'Hagan, Divis, & Long, 2008; SAMHSA, 2005). The method of preventing combative behavior can begin with gathering information about triggers and what works to prevent escalation, or help the patient to feel safe (SAMHSA, 2005). Steps provided throughout the training program, are designed to strengthen the organization with guidance, explore coping mechanisms, decrease mental health stigma, increase education about seclusion or the use of restraints, prevention methods and personal behavior modification or techniques (SAMHSA, 2005).

The benefit of using the education and literature on seclusion and restraints for this education project, is that it offers support and addresses the need for preventing escalation and how to decrease incidences of violence. The next article discusses best practices to eliminate restraints and seclusion; with a spotlight on workforce development, staff education, promote patient autonomy, escalation prevention with early intervention tools, and debriefing (O'Hagan, Divis, & Long, 2008). Highlighting the prevention and debriefing sections from this article as planning and re-evaluation of the methods or approach is vital to improve the outcome for the patient. Several plans and assessments can be employed to predict the rise of behavior escalation with knowledge specific to the patient, to ensure escalation is prevented with a blueprint of what works for the patient. The debriefing is used as a tool for staff to reconfigure what should be done better and offered as a learning opportunity. Additional benefits of the debriefing help staff to share how they feel about the experience and areas where they feel improvements should be made (O'Hagan, Divis, & Long, 2008).

Local Background and Context

When the mental health units are filled in the hospital, the emergency room will stabilize the patient and refer them to a local mental health and recovery center. The setting for this doctoral project is located Orlando, Florida, in a small private mental health and recovery center; that accepts insured patients who are suffering from mental illness and substance abuse. In this setting, there will be approximately 25 staff members that would be a target for this education program. On a monthly average, the facility admits "85 patients with 30 that are or have volatile tendencies, with most having a criminal history" (K. Alexander, personal communication, January 22, 2019). Currently, the facility does not have an education program to help prevent violence escalation. At this present time, the federal government does not have workplace violence protections in place; and the Occupational Safety and Health Administration (OSHA) only have recommendations for healthcare agencies to report violent episodes (Trinkoff et al., n.d.). Despite the recovery center reporting "eight verbal and one physical escalation last month, there has been a steady increase of volatile admissions over the last few months" (K. Alexander, personal communication, January 22, 2019). The facility management expressed a need for an education program, as there has been an increase of verbal escalation leading to a recent physical attack on a nurse.

Role of the Doctor of Nursing Practice Student

Currently, I am a nursing professor at an area school of nursing, teaching didactic, lab, and clinical for a registered nursing (RN) program in the Orlando area. My affiliation with the recovery center is clinical and project-based for this project. Potential personal bias with this project is that nurses may not consider the impact of not reporting violent situations, and how it can directly affect nursing safety. My role with this doctoral project is to create an education program geared toward preventing behavior escalation and decreasing violent incidents in the healthcare unit. Once the education was created with the facility experts, my role then was to create an education presentation with coordinating hand-outs for future use of this education program.

Role of the Project Team

When determining the success of this doctoral project, it was vital to consider the roles of those chosen. The interdisciplinary team consisted of a physician, FNP, and a staff nurse, all of whom are experts in their field. The nurses have been in the field for a combined 50 years. The physician has been in the profession for approximately 25 years and has valuable expertise with mental health, mental illness, and addiction. The collective experience of the project team involves knowledge of addiction therapy, behavior modification, acute and chronic mental illness. Each expert involved in the creation of this project brought their observations of past or current situations of verbal or physical escalation. My role was to determine the gap in practice and lead the team by performing the review of literature and developing the education program.

When I concluded the project with the interdisciplinary team of experts, they received the created staff education materials, hand-outs to assist in the teaching program, and the education evaluation form. During the final stages of transferring the project to the facility, the team was consulted with the creation of a plan to implement the completed project. Within 3-months of the completion of this project, the Director of Nursing will hand the materials over to the education specialist for evaluation. In 6months, the training program will be administered to all nursing staff. The goal is to prevent escalation of violent encounters with combative patients.

Summary

The purpose of this project was to develop an education program for nursing staff regarding strategies to prevent escalation of violent behavior in combative patients. The gap in practice is that nurses are not prepared to prevent violence escalation, due to the lack of knowledge of how to work with combative patients. Concepts utilized for this staff education project stem from the social cognitive theory, and adaptation theory, which were applied to create evidence-based education regarding strategies to prevent escalation of violence. Once the project was completed, the materials were handed over to the facility to implement into their long-term education program.

Section 3: Collection and Analysis of Evidence

Introduction

The ANA (2018) #EndNurseAbuse survey revealed out of 14,000 nurses who responded, 62% stated they had suffered both physical and verbal abuse from patients. Violence is affecting nurses in various ways, from burn-out to post-traumatic stress disorder, resulting in low morale, productivity, an increase of call-offs and turnover (Gates, Gillespie, & Succop, 2011). The project site is a recovery center inpatient facility with outpatient programs that focus on those who are seeking help for substance abuse and mental illness. The team of experts within the facility agreed with the project focus on an education program regarding violence escalation in combative patients for nursing staff.

The purpose of this project was to develop an education program for nursing staff regarding strategies to prevent escalation of violent behavior in combative patients. The next section will review the practice-focus question, sources of evidence, and an analysis and synthesis of pertinent information relating to this project. Nurses play a large, intricate role in the process of care of all patients, in every capacity and situation. Not having the information needed through either a formal education setting or continuing facility education to help nurses understand how to holistically care for combative and combative patients; could leave both experienced and new nurses open for mental or physical injury. The goal is to prevent escalation of violent encounters with combative patients.

Practice-Focus Question

The local problem is that the selected urban hospital's leadership has recognized the need to provide additional education for staff to improve their nursing staff's ability to work with combative patients and prevent escalation of violence. The gap in practice is that nurses are not prepared to prevent violence escalation, due to the lack of knowledge of how to work with combative patients. The guiding question for this project was: Will an education program for nurses working with potentially combative patients increase their knowledge of strategies to prevent escalation of violent behavior? When nurses do not have the knowledge or resources to assist them with learning how to work with patients who exhibit combative behavior, they have a high incidence of becoming a victim of abuse (Taylor, 1983). The purpose of this project was to develop an education program for nursing staff regarding strategies to prevent escalation of violent behavior in combative patients.

Sources of Evidence

The project education program was developed based on published literature in combination with valuable input from the project team, consisting of a physician, FNP, and a staff nurse. The team of experts employed for this project were well-rounded, established within their fields, have valuable insight, and working knowledge of common deficiencies when caring for a potentially volatile patient. The team of experts have a combined experience of over 50 years and agreed that an education program would be beneficial to their facility.

The guiding question for this project was: Will an education program for nurses working with potentially combative patients increase their knowledge of strategies to prevent escalation of violent behavior? The education development was guided by social cognitive theory, created by Albert Bandura, which describes how personal experiences, behavioral patterns, life events, and environmental factors influence the outcome of an event (Bandura, 2001). Nurses may or may not understand the concept of how modeling behavior could benefit their outcome with the nurse-patient relationship (Sidhu & Park, 2018). If the nurse does not recognize the need for an outlet to cope with the on-going stressful events of the healthcare environment, it can lead to compassion fatigue, burnout, and post-traumatic stress disorder, reducing the ability to adapt (Schmidt & Haglund, 2017). As a result, the behavior escalation prevention education program can assist in the reduction of workplace injuries, enabling the nurse to enhance their well-being and gain mastery with working in potentially volatile patient scenarios (Chapman et al., 2010).

Program Development

As a part of the ethical protection of the project team of experts, each individual voluntarily participated in the development of the education program and was allowed to withdraw at any time. This educational project was required to be submitted through the Walden University Institutional Review Board (IRB) for ethics approval, and to comply with the site facility IRB policies and procedures. To locate relevant literature to synthesize information for the educational program, I used the CINAHL, MEDLINE, and the Joanna Briggs Institute databases. Keywords used for the search included *violence against nurses, patient on nurse violence, de-escalation, education programs, burn-out, posttraumatic stress disorder, workplace violence, mental illness, mental health, social cognitive theory, adaptation theory, behavior prevention education programs, physical violence, verbal abuse, reporting* workplace violence, strategies for de-escalation, addiction, and anxiety. Articles over 15 years were discarded, though sources about psychology theories/theorists range up to 35 years.

Analysis and Synthesis

The content obtained through a literature search was instrumental in the creation of the escalation behavior prevention program. The initial draft of the education program was developed from the gathered literature. To ensure the project remains on track, it was vital for my role as the project manager to present the details to the team for discussion. It was the project manager's responsibility to incorporate the team's feedback regarding the initial draft into a revision of the education and present the revision to the team for review. At the conclusion of the project, all deliverables were handed over to the facility for later implementation. Deliverables were defined as education materials, associated handouts, a plan for education delivery and evaluation of learning. Once the project was complete, the team of experts provided project evaluation through a survey regarding their satisfaction with the planning process and the leadership provided by myself. See Appendix A for the questionnaire that was used for the project evaluation.

Summary

The purpose of this project was to develop an education program for nursing staff regarding strategies to prevent escalation of violent behavior in combative patients. After a review of the literature, an education program was developed for nurses that are working in a mental health and recovery center. The goal is to prevent escalation of violent encounters with combative patients. This program included educational materials and hand-outs to help nurses remember the reviewed material. An evaluation form was developed and was included for subsequent use to evaluate the participants learning. The planning team of experts provided project evaluation through a survey regarding their satisfaction with the planning process.

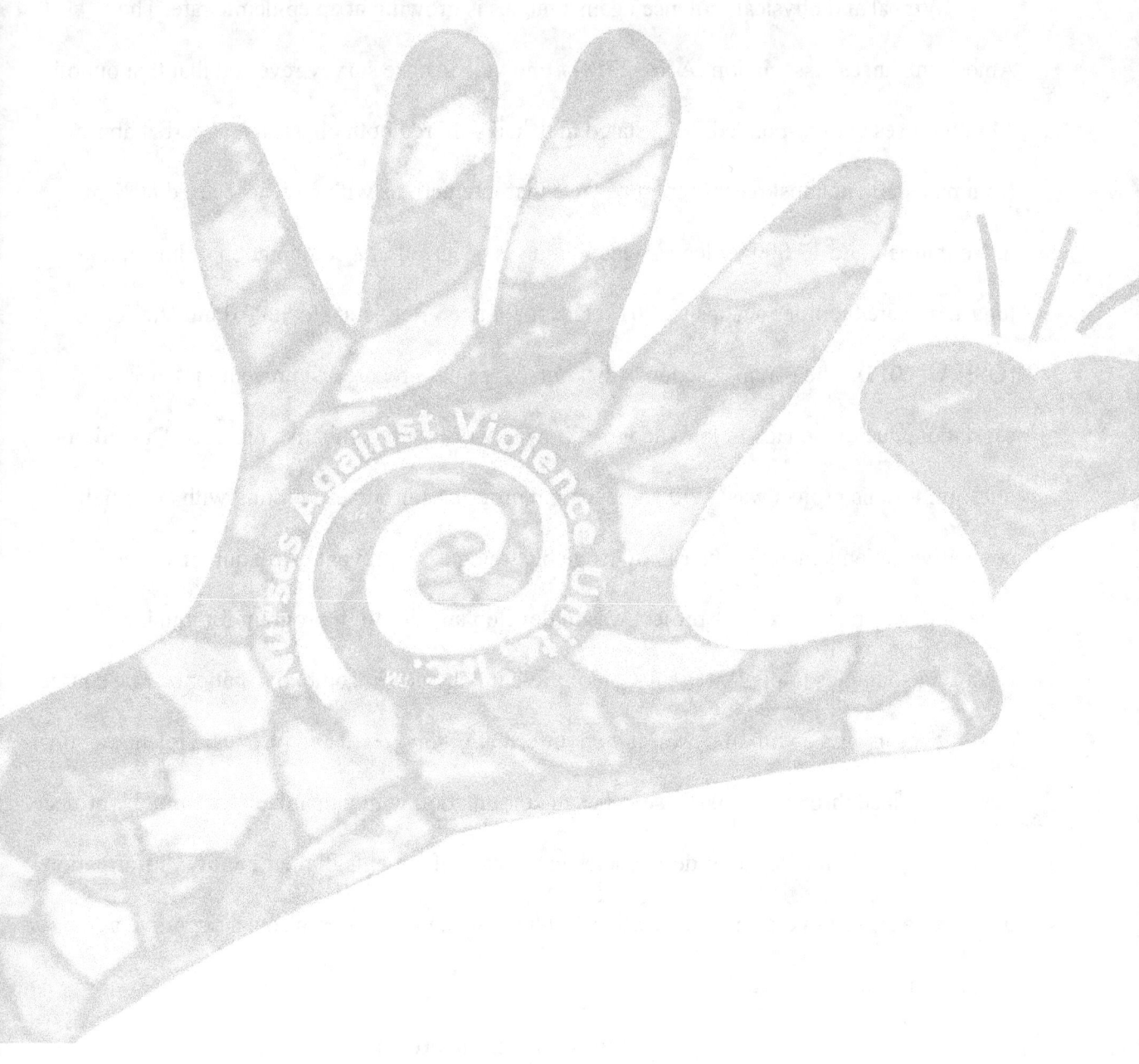

Section 4: Findings and Recommendations

Introduction

Verbal and physical violence against nurses is growing at an epidemic rate. The American Nurses Association (ANA,2018) #EndNurseAbuse survey revealed that that out of 14,000 nurses who responded, 62% stated they had suffered both physical and verbal abuse from patients. The most recent report reflects that interactions with patients caused 80% of nurse injuries, and 17,000 violence-related injuries occurred in a combination of hospital and long-term care facilities (Esposito, 2017, Occupational Safety and Health Administration [OSHA], 2015). The gap in practice is that nurses are not prepared to prevent violence escalation, due to the lack of knowledge of how to work with combative patients. The guiding question for this project was: Will an education program for nurses working with potentially combative patients increase their knowledge of strategies to prevent escalation of violent behavior? The purpose of this project was to develop an education program for nursing staff regarding strategies to prevent escalation of violent behavior in combative patients. The sources of evidence involved with this project were information on verbal and physical violence against nurses obtained through scholarly searches in combination with valuable input from the project team of experts' knowledge of deficiencies in the care of patients in their facility. Information gathered was used to create the education and handouts, utilizing both social cognitive and adaptation theories.

Findings and Implications

Findings from the literature review that were included in this project are; awareness, recognizing the beginning symptoms of behavior escalation, implementing conflict resolution with increased communication, and the benefits of debriefing (Forster et al., 1999; Johansen, 2012; NASMHPD, 2006; SAMHSA, 2005). Other areas covered in this program include the creation of a safe environment for the nurse to express feelings, report violent events, and increase both interprofessional and interprofessional communication. A draft of the educational program was created and distributed to the project team of experts for review and further input. The team of experts included a physician, a FNP, and a staff nurse who currently work on a mental health and recovery unit. The team of experts was given a timeline at the beginning of the project, and quarterly to reveal progress. During the first meeting, the team discussed the educational objectives. The objectives identified for the escalation behavior prevention program synthesized from the gathered literature were:

1. Review situations that could potentially increase patient stress levels.
2. Recognize the beginning symptoms of behavior escalation.
3. Review conflict resolution and the need for communication.
4. Recognize the importance of self-care and reporting events.

Team meetings were guided by the objectives and organized into short, simple steps with rationales for simple knowledge assimilation. Team discussions focused on a three-step approach to escalation prevention. The first step is awareness, which consists of reviewing the patient's situation, support system, and employment, while observing their actions and reactions. Awareness must also include understanding of the patient's commitment status (voluntary or involuntarily), their use of substances, and decisions regarding further assessment criteria. The second step is prevention, through reflection on the patient's behavior and possible explanations such as flashbacks undiagnosed or untreated. The third and final step is conflict resolution, in which the nurse helps the patient through a difficult moment with increased therapeutic communication. The team discussed these specific behavior techniques:

1. Recognize stress behaviors.
2. Address the issue before the loss of control.
3. Actively listen, using non-verbal and verbal communication methods.
4. Be aware of one's breathing and slow it down.
5. Identify the problem and find a solution.

The last area that ties the three steps together is debriefing and reporting the event. Without reporting the verbal or physical incident, the facility is unaware of the trauma created for the staff member. Mandatory debriefing measures are suggested to help prevent staffing issues by increasing the milieu and remaining cognizant of the noise stimulation on the unit.

A draft education presentation was discussed in the second team meeting. During the final meeting, the team critiqued and revised educational handouts, to ensure their coordination with the information on the presentation and effectiveness to promote recall of the escalation behavior prevention program, and subsequent training. The team of experts remained in sync with one another and were successful in planning assistance by sharing input, insight, and experiences needed to create the escalation prevention program.

The project site received a visit from their accreditation organization during the same approximate time that team meetings for planning the project education program had been scheduled. The accreditation visit created unexpected fluctuations in the team's schedules, which was resolved through virtual and in-person meetings to ensure deadlines met the demands of this project. When the accreditation review was completed with remediations resolved, in-person meetings resumed as scheduled.

At the conclusion of the staff education project, the team of three experts completed an evaluation questionnaire located in Appendix A. All members answered agree or strongly agree that the problem was clear, and the literature was analyzed and synthesized to reflect the need for staff education to prevent violence escalation in the workplace. One of the evaluators mentioned in their evaluation that staff nurses expressed that they would feel more confident and ready to work with patients to prevent combative behavior if there was a program in place. The team of experts all agreed that the project objective to develop and create an education program that will focus on strategies to prevent escalation of violent behavior for nurses has been met. Every member in the team of experts agreed that I had exhibited leadership throughout the project; the flow was organized, and scheduled meetings were on-time and efficient. The team of experts were happy about the staff education program, as it gives valuable information to fill in gaps of knowledge that the nurse will need to keep themselves and others safe in the workplace.

Education on preventing violence escalation is essential for nurses that work with patients that potentially may be volatile. The concept of escalation prevention decreases the need for de-escalation techniques; through being more aware, recognizing increased stress, conflict resolution with increased communication, and the benefits of debriefing. When a patient reaches the point of escalation, their voice becomes elevated, verbally abusive and at times resulting in physical attacks. The concept behind de-escalation is to subdue and control a patient that has reached a level of behavior escalation that is combative and puts the patient, other patients, and nursing staff at risk for injury. Whereas, an escalation prevention program gives the nurse tools to recognize signs of increased stress, to help the patient calm down which ultimately will prevent further escalation. Eventually, the nurse will become proficient in escalation prevention skills and become resilient in protecting their mental and physical health (Chapman et al., 2010; Taylor, 1983).

There are many implications that can arise from having an escalation prevention program in place. Staff nurses who receive this prevention training will have new and updated information to help them understand how to care for someone who is in mental health or addiction crisis and develop better understanding of self-care and coping mechanisms to protect themselves from absorbing the behaviors on the unit. For individuals in the community, nurses who are utilizing the escalation behavior prevention program will ultimately assist the patient in having a more holistic approach to their care, reducing the incidence of increasing trauma to the patient and nurse. The recovery center may benefit from an escalation prevention program through improved staff satisfaction, reduced nurse turnover and workforce shortages. Financial benefit to the facility is possible if patient satisfaction measures increase, which then trigger improved reimbursement from insurance carriers. When the initial draft was presented, all members responded with positive feedback and stated that the information created was relevant to the current trends in healthcare and promoted social change.

Recommendations

The gap in practice is that nurses are not prepared to prevent violence escalation, due to the lack of knowledge of how to work with combative patients. The staff education program covers the topics of preventing behavior escalation by covering the gap in practice through increasing knowledge, awareness, symptom recognition, conflict resolution with communication, and debriefing of the event. Added benefits of the education project will give the nurse tools for success to prevent injuries and mental trauma from the event. The completed project includes the educational program in an electronic presentation, one handout, and a questionnaire that will evaluate the understanding of the learned material.

The electronic presentation (Appendix B) will contain 13 slides that will cover the steps of the escalation behavior prevention program in detail. It was important to align the steps of the education program in the handout, keep it simple, and easy to read as a summary of the strategies for the nurse on-the-go. (see Appendix C). The escalation prevention education will be delivered in-person by a trained expert, with attendance mandatory for all RNs working on the mental health and recovery units. New employees will receive the education during orientation as preparation for working with potentially volatile patients. Subsequently, RNs will independently review the electronic presentation during their annual training and complete the comprehensive questionnaire as evaluation of learning.

Appendix D contains the comprehension questionnaire, to be completed before and after the education. Six multiple choice questions are designed to evaluate learning. The comprehension questionnaire also contains space for the participants to offer suggestions if they choose, which can assist the organization with future updates of the educational material. When the project concluded, the team of experts had all the education materials to begin their escalation prevention education program for the nurses. Implementation of the escalation prevention education program could help decrease violent encounters with combative patients and result in less escalation of violence when encounters do occur.

Contributions of the Doctoral Project Team

The team of experts used for this doctoral project consisted of a medical physician, nurse practitioner, and a staff nurse who work in the mental health and recovery units. I selected these leaders to assist with the creation of the educational program due to their experience working with volatile patients, and their ability to ensure all nurses utilize the training for the safety of patients and staff. The team of experts were supportive and forthcoming with providing information that would lead to the discovery of the gap in practice and feedback on the education that was created. Although not a psychiatrist, the physician has spent over 25 years working patients' mental health and addiction problems, experiencing how certain patients may get triggered in a healthcare setting if the nurse is not adequately prepared through education or training. The FNP was instrumental in guiding the facility-specific details and how the education could be specifically applied in the project facility. Finally, I observed nurse-patient interactions while shadowing the staff nurse, who also assisted with the project by soliciting nurses' views about the current events of potentially volatile situations. Over some time, the use of the program evaluations and comments/suggestions area will help the team of experts with updating the escalation prevention education. When working in a facility that does not have continuing education on managing combative patient encounters, the escalation prevention education program can be the missing link to build strong education to help nurses keep patients and staff members safe.

Strengths and Limitations of the Project

The local problem is that the selected urban hospital's leadership has recognized the need to provide additional education for staff to improve their nursing staff's ability to work with combative patients and prevent escalation. There are many strengths to this education project. When conducting a literature review, many articles supported the need for an escalation prevention education program for nurses. The main strength of this program is the welcome and participation from the facility to develop an education program that will be utilized in their facility to enhance safety on the units. Some nurses have preconceived barriers about working with patients that are potentially volatile, which is a limitation of the education developed during this project. It is important to eliminate preconceived ideas of mental health and addiction, also known as stigma, as it can lead to patient behavior escalation if the nurse is not adequately trained.

Section 5: Dissemination Plan

Dissemination Plan

The purpose of this project was to develop an education program for nursing staff regarding strategies to prevent escalation of violent behavior in combative patients. The goal for dissemination in the small mental health and recovery center will be simple as it is a stand-alone facility and the planning team of experts received the education and will distribute it to the Director of Nursing for decision regarding delivery to nursing staff. There are other means of dissemination for this education project, and this is to promote the use and benefits through social media, share project findings in professional conferences for nurses and healthcare leadership, publication in a journal, and write a book. There are various organizations that I would like to disseminate this valuable information to would include American Nurse Today, Journal of Forensic Nursing,

Journal of Psychiatric and Mental Health Nursing, Journal of Nursing Education, and Nursing Standard. Some of these journals are linked to professional organizations that hold yearly conferences and may have the opportunity to submit my project for publication. There also may be an opportunity to speak and discuss the need for a program to prevent violent behavior and decrease violence in the workplace.

Analysis of Self

Throughout my DNP program, I was allowed to improve the care of both patients and nurses through various roles as a scholar, practitioner, and project manager. As a scholar, I have excelled within my field of developing an education program aimed to decrease and prevent violence escalation. Working as a practitioner within the nursing field, I can relate to the material, and bring my knowledge to create a viable education program. Using the AACN (2016) DNP essential VI: Interprofessional collaboration for improving patient and population outcomes, it aligns with the role of a project manager. Working with the team of experts, through interprofessional communication, we were able to locate the gap in practice and complete this project seamlessly. The increased communication and professionalism were a determining factor for the success of this project.

The completion of the project was both a challenging and rewarding experience. As a nurse leader, it is essential to slow down and observe all aspects of issues leading to a greater problem. The challenge was determining from the nursing quality indicators a possible issue. Instead, I found the connection between staffing, nursing turnover, job satisfaction, and psychiatric physical abuse (Montalvo, 2007). Through the brainstorming and development of the project, it has expanded my knowledge and expertise within my profession. I have grown into a nurse leader, pausing to reflect, listening to feedback, and incorporating valuable ideas into my practice. Long-term professional goals include but not limited to public speaking, training seminars, build more programs to help nurses, and continue to expand my knowledge.

Summary

The purpose of this project is to develop an education program for nursing staff regarding strategies to prevent escalation of violent behavior in combative patients. The gap in practice was discovered that nurses are not prepared to prevent violence escalation, due to the lack of knowledge of how to work with combative patients. Collaborating with the interprofessional team of experts, we were able to develop an education program aimed to increase knowledge regarding strategies to prevent escalation of violence when working with combative patients. Upon the completion of the educational project, the mental health and recovery center received the complete escalation prevention education program, consisting of an electronic presentation, handout, and a comprehension questionnaire for evaluation of learning. The knowledge gained through this education program will help prepare nurses recognize the beginning stages of stress and use strategies to prevent escalation behavior, with the goal to decrease escalation of violence when working with combative patients. The improved culture of safety that results will bring a potential for positive social change for both nurses and the patients under their care.

Appendix A: Evaluation Questionnaire for Team of Experts

Stakeholder/Team Member Evaluation of DNP Project

Problem:

Purpose:

Goal:

Objective:

Scale: SD=Strongly Disagree   D=Disagree   U=Uncertain   A=Agree   SA=Strongly Agree

	1=SD	2=D	3=UC	4=A	SA=5
Q1 Was the problem made clear to you in the beginning?	___	___	___	___	___
Q2 Did the DNP student analyze and synthesize the literature for the team?	___	___	___	___	___ evidence-based
Q3 Was the stated program goal appropriate?	___	___	___	___	___
Q4 Was the stated project objective met?	___	___	___	___	___ Q5 How would you rate the DNP student's leadership throughout the process?	___	___	___	___	___
Q6 Were meeting agendas sent out in a timely manner?	___	___	___	___	___ Q7 Were meeting minutes submitted in a timely manner?	___	___	___	___	___
Q8 Were meetings held to the allotted time frame?	___	___	___	___	___
Q9 Would you consider the meetings productive?	___	___	___	___	___
Q10 Do you feel that you had input into the process?	___	___	___	___	___

Q11 Please comment on areas where you feel the DNP student excelled or might learn from your advice/suggestions:

Appendix B: Behavior Prevention Educational Program

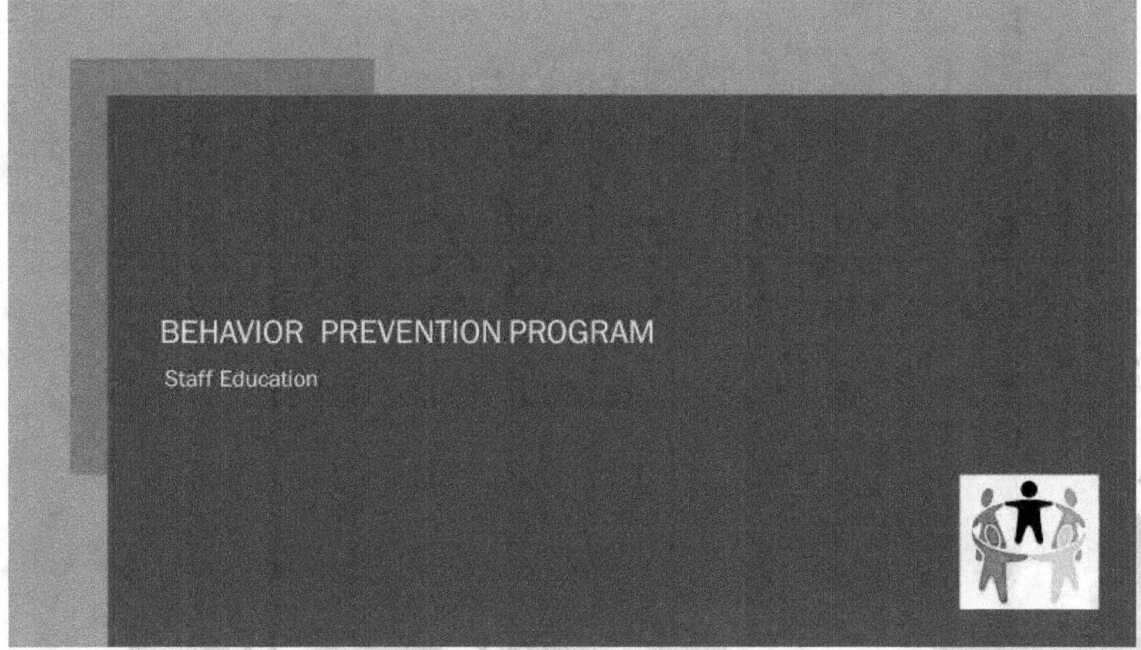

Behavior Prevention Program: Staff Education

Objectives:

This presentation on violence prevention will educate nurses to stay safe while working with potentially volatile patients in our mental health and recovery areas.

This presentation will:

- Review situations that could potentially increase patient stress levels.
- Recognize beginning symptoms of behavior escalation.
- Review conflict resolution and the need for communication.
- Recognize the importance of self-care and reporting events.

1st Step to Prevention:
Awareness

- The 1st step to preventing escalation is being Aware of patient's situation.
    - When obtaining a history, it is vital to find out where the patient is living, if they have any family or support system.
    - Do they have a job?
    - Are they using substances? What kind? The last time used?
    - Are they using medication to control their impulses and mood?
    - How is the patient acting?
    - Another area to explore is the decrease of behavior triggers and risk for violence (NASMHPD, 2006).

1st Step to Prevention:
Awareness & Understanding the Patient

- Upon admission: Situational Anxiety – Fear of the unknown.
- Patients may have an undiagnosed or diagnosed mental illness.
- Patient may be medicated or unmedicated.
- Baker Acted – BA52 Involuntary 72-hour hold, pending a Psych Evaluation.
- Addiction, possible withdrawals
- Homeless

1st Step to Prevention:
Awareness

- While assessing and obtaining information from the patient, the social cognitive theory (SCT) addresses personal life experiences, life events, behavioral patterns, mixed with environmental factors interact with another, influencing each other (Bandura, 2001).

- Beliefs play a role in how a patient is perceived during the assessment and the behavior that may arise throughout their stay (Bandura, 1989).

- It has been suggested that behavior that is exhibited from nurses or patients may model one's behavior or actions (Sidhu & Park, 2018).

2nd Step to Prevention:
Recognizing Escalation

The patient may show anxiety or increased stress level by pacing, short abrupt answers, looking around, no eye contact, rubbing hands together, and talking louder then before.
Verbal escalation may start at this point.

- Several things may be happening to the patient:
  - Has a psychiatric condition either diagnosed or undiagnosed
  - Addiction issues, possible withdrawals
  - No support system
  - Childcare issues
  - Money worries
  - Afraid

3rd Step to Prevention:
Conflict Resolution

Ensure the patient's safety and privacy. — Ex: The patient is admitted to a unit, and may be scared.

↓

Ask if there is someone that you can contact for the patient. — Ex: The patient may need help finding someone to get their children from school.

↓

Get into the patient's world — Taking a minute as hard as it could be can really make a difference to someone upset.

3rd Step to Prevention:
Conflict Resolution

- **Scenario:**

    Patient arrived to the unit about 15 minutes prior to your shift, they are looking around, isolating themselves from the rest of the patients. Their body is sitting straight and you see them repeatedly shaking their leg. You just briefly noticed this person may be upset yet, you need to organize your day. The patient gets up and walks to the nurses station and starts raising their voice stating they want to leave.

    Question: What would the staff member do first?

3rd Step to Prevention:
Conflict Resolution & Increase Communication

Answer: Stop what you are doing! Take a few minutes to talk with the patient and see how you can help them.

Something to consider, if the patient is homeless, off of their medication and showing physical signs of stress, then the first thing that should be done is bring them to a quiet place, then offer something to eat or drink.

3rd Step to Prevention:
Conflict Resolution & Self-Preservation

The Combined Steps to Prevent Injury:

- Be aware and recognize increased stress behaviors.
- Address the issue before the patient has lost control.
- Actively listen, exercising verbal and non-verbal communication methods.
- Watch your breathing, slow it down.
- Identify the problem and find a solution (Johansen, 2012).

Debriefing

- Immediately hold Debriefing After the Event.
- Notify the Supervisor of the Event.
- Top Organization, Supervisors, and Support Staff meet within 24-48 hours following the Event (NASMHPD, 2006).

Debriefing

- Everyone involved in a hostile situation will need to debrief.
    - *To identify anything that created the patient to start escalating.*
        - Revise their plan of care.
        - Increase the milieu of the unit.
        - Staffing issues
        - Noise, increased environmental stimuli (NASMHPD, 2006).

Debriefing

- To ensure those involved feel supported.
    - *Identify coping mechanisms for Nursing Staff*
        - Exercise
        - Laughing
        - Traveling
    - *Were holistic methods of coping taught to the patient?*
        - Guided Imagery
        - Meditation
        - Voluntary time out (SAMHSA, 2005).

Appendix C: Education Handout

Behavior Prevention Education Handout

1st Step of Prevention: Awareness

Consider what the patient is going through. Questions to ask yourself:

1) Are they homeless?
2) Do they have a history of a violent past?
3) How is the patient acting?
4) Have they been involuntarily committed?
5) Does the patient use drugs or alcohol?
6) History of psychiatric illness? Treated? Untreated?

2nd Step of Prevention: Recognizing Escalation

Signs to look for:

1) Does the patient appear to be isolating themselves?
2) Pacing
3) Fidgeting
4) Looking around, appearing to look unsure or nervous.
5) Poor eye contact
6) Short abrupt answers, voice is getting louder.

3rd Step of Prevention: Conflict Resolution

1) Be aware and recognize increased stress behaviors.
2) Address the issue before the patient has lost control.
3) Actively listen, verbally and non-verbally
4) Watch your breathing, slow it down.
5) Solve the problem.

Debriefing

> Immediately Hold a Debriefing After the Event → Notify the Supervisor if they have not been notified already. → Top Organization, Supervisors, and Support Staff meet within 24-48 hours following the Event.

Remember Self-Care! When you can, exercise, meditate, laugh, take a fun trip, take breaks & Eat!

Appendix D: Educational Program Comprehension Questionnaire

Behavior Prevention Education Program: Comprehension Questionnaire

Name:_____

Supervisor:_____

1) The behavior prevention education program is designed to help prevent the patient from getting upset or angry.   True or False

2) It is important for the nurse to review or ask questions about work, living situations, and family support. Why?
   a. To see if you are related.
   b. To alert a social worker to help patient to feel more at ease.
   c. The patient may want assistance and is either too afraid to ask or they do not know they exist.

3) Can you interchange the steps of prevention?
   a. Yes. One can happen before the other.
   b. No. They are stuck and have to be in sequence.

4) Social cognitive theory is the way we perceive our environment and how one interacts with another.   True or False

5) What are signs of elevated stress?
   a. No eye contact
   b. Rubbing hands together
   c. Raised voice level
   d. All of the Above

6) Can nurses absorb the behavior from the environment?   True or False

Comments or Suggestions:

References

Adams, J., Roddy, A., Knowles, A., Ashworth, J., & Irons, G. (n.d.). Assessing the effectiveness of clinical educationto reduce the frequency and recurrence of workplace violence. *Austrialian Journal of Advanced Nursing, 34*, 6-15.

Advisory Board. (2016, May 3). Nearly 75 percent of all workplace assaults happen in health care, researchers find. *The Daily Briefing*.

Agency for Healthcare Research and Quality. (2016). Grant application basics. Retrieved from https://www.ahrq.gov/funding/process/grant-app-basics/index.html

Agency for Healthcare Research and Quality. (2016). *Strategies to de-escalate aggressive behavior in psychiatric patients* (180). Retrieved from https://effectivehealthcare.ahrq.gov/sites/default/files/related_files/aggression_executive.pdf

American Association of Colleges of Nursing. (2006). *The essentials of doctoral education for advanced nursing practice*. Retrieved from ACCN Nursing website: http://www.aacnnursing.org/Education-Resources/AACN-Essentials

American College of Emergency Physicians. (2009). Emergency Department Violence. Retrieved from http://newsroom.acep.org/2009-01-04-emergency-department-violence-fact-sheet

American Nurses Association. (2018, April 18). ANA responds to the Joint Commission sentinal event alert on physical and verbal violence against healthcare workers. *Nursing World*.

Angland, S., Dowling, M., & Casey, D. (2013, September 20). Nurses' perceptions of the factors which cause violence and aggression in the emergency department: A qualitative study. *International Emergency Nursing, 22*, 134-139. http://dx.doi.org/http://dx.doi.org/10.1016/j.ienj.2013.09.005

Arnetz, J. E., Hamblin, L., Ager, J., Aranyos, D., Essenmacher, L., Upfal, M. J., & Luborsky, M. (2013, October 12). Using database reports to reduce workplace violence: Perceptions of hospital stakeholders. *Work, 51*, 51-59.

Arnetz, J. E., Hamblin, L., Ager, J., Luborsky, M., Upfal, M. J., Russell, J., & Essenmacher, L. (2015, May). Underreporting of Workplace Violence. *Workplace Health & Safety*, 200-210. http://dx.doi.org/10.1177/2165079915574684

Ashton, R. A., Morris, L., & Smith, I. (2017, December 20). A qualitative meta-synthesis of emergency department staff experiences of violence and aggression. *International Emergency Nursing, 39*, 13-19. http://dx.doi.org/https://doi.org/10.1016/j.ienj.2017.12.004

Bandura, A. (1989, September). Human agency in social cognitive theory. *American Psychologist, 44*, 1175-1184.

Bandura, A. (2001). Social cognitive theory: An agentic perspective. *Annual Review Psychology, 52*, 1-26.

Bandura, A. (2010, June 22). *Bandura's Social Cognitive Theory: An Introduction* [Video file]. Retrieved from https://www.youtube.com/watch?v=S4N5J9jFW5U

Bolvin, J. M. (2018, November). 2018 Nursing trends and salary results. *American Nurse Today*, *13*(11).

Bowers, L., Nijman, H., Allan, T., Simpson, A., Warren, J., & Turner, L. (2006, June). Prevention and management of aggression training and violent incidents on U.K. acute psychiatric wards. *Psychiatric Services*, *57*, 1022-1026.

Bowman, S. (2013). Impact on electronic health record systems on information integrity: Quality and safety implications. Retrieved from https://www.ncbi.nlm.nih.gov/pmc/articles/PMC3797550/

Brent, N. J. (2016, November 11). Nursing careers and jobs [Blog post]. Retrieved from https://www.nurse.com/blog/2016/11/11/how-nurses-can-help-reduce-their-patients-anxiety/

Bureau of Labor Statistics. (2012, February). The recession of 2007-2009. *BLS spotlight on statistics*, 1-18. Retrieved from https://www.bls.gov/spotlight/2012/recession/pdf/recession_bls_spotlight.pdf

Chapman, R., Styles, I., Perry, L., & Combs, S. (2010). Nurses' experience of adjusting to workplace violence: A theory of adaptation. *International Journal of Mental Health Nursing*, *19*, 186-194. http://dx.doi.org/10.1111/j.1447-0349.2009.00663.x

Chen, W., Huang, C., Hwang, J., & Chen, C. (2010, June 10). The relationship of health-related quality of life to workplace physical violence against nurses by psychiatric patients. *Quality of Life Research*, *19*, 1155-1161. http://dx.doi.org/10.1007/s11136-010-9679-4

Chen, W., Huang, C., Hwang, J., & Chen, C. (2010, May 17). The relationship of health-related quality of life to workplace physical violence against nurses by psychiatric patients. *Quality of Life Research*, *19*, 1155-1161. http://dx.doi.org/10.1007/s11136-010-9679-4

Chojnacka, F. T. (2005, February 3). Reporting incidents of violence and aggression towards NHS staff. *Nursing Standard*, *19*, 51-56.

Coleman, C. (2015, June). Stimulating a culture of improvement: Introducing an integrated quality tool for organizational self-assessment. *Clinical Journal of Oncology Nursing*, *19*, 261-264. http://dx.doi.org/10.1188/15.CJON.261-264

Colvin, & Sugai (1989). Stages of behavior escalation. Retrieved from https://k12engagement.unl.edu/Stages%20of%20Behavior%20Escalation.pdf

Communication 5: Effective listening and observation skills [Discussion comment]. (2018, March 12). Retrieved from https://www.nursingtimes.net/clinical-archive/assessment-skills/communication-5-effective-listening-and-observation-skills/7023622.article

Copeland, D., & Henry, M. (2017, April). Workplace violence and perceptions of safety among emergency department staff members: Experiences, expectations, tolerance, reporting, and recommendations. *Journal of Trauma Nursing*, *24*, 65-77, E1-E2.

de Carvalho, E. C., Oliveiro-Kumakura, A. R., & Vasconcelos Morais, S. C. (2016, April 12). Clinical reasoning in nursing: Teaching strategies and assessment tools. *Revista Brasileira de Enfermagem*, *70*, 662-667. http://dx.doi.org/http://dx.doi.org/10.1590/0034-7167-2016-0509

DeMarco, M., & Tilson, E. R. (n.d.). Maslow in the classroom and the clinic. *Teaching Techniques*, *70*, 91-94.

Department of Health and Human Services. (1999). *Mental health: A report of the surgeon general* [Report]. Retrieved from https://profiles.nlm.nih.gov/ps/access/NNBBHS.pdf

Department of Mental Health Law & Policy. (2014). *Baker Act; The Florida Mental Health Act* [User reference guide]. Retrieved from http://www.dcf.state.fl.us/programs/samh/mentalhealth/laws/BakerActManual.pdf

Djulbegovic, B. (2014). A framework to bridge the gaps between evidence-based medicine, health outcomes, and improvement and implementation science. *Journal of Oncology Practice*, *10*, 200-202.

Doody, C. M., & Doody, O. (2011, May). Introducing evidence into nursing practice: using the Iowa model. *British Journal of Nursing*, *20*, 661-664.

DuBose, J. R., & Hadi, K. (2016, November 10). Improving inpatient environments to support patient sleep. *International Journal for Quality in Health Care*, *28*, 540-553. http://dx.doi.org/https://doi.org/10.1093/intqhc/mzw079

Esposito, L. (2017). Nurses face more violence from hospital patients. Retrieved from https://health.usnews.com/wellness/articles/2017-01-18/nurses-face-more-violence-from-hospital-patients

Fawcett, J., & Garity, J. (2009). Chapter 1: Research and evidence-based nursing practice. *Evaluating Research for Evidence-Based Nursing*, 3-20.

Florida Council for Community Mental Health. (2011, January). Mentally ill individuals use of emergency departments: Fact sheet. *Florida Council for Community Mental Health*. Retrieved from http://www.fccmh.org/resources/docs/Emergency_Departments.pdf

Florida Department of Children and Families. (2014). Baker Act involuntary examination criteria, processes and timeframes. Retrieved from https://www.dcf.state.fl.us/programs/samh/MentalHealth/laws/bainvex.pdf

Florida Department of Education. (2018). *PSAV Programs; Practical Nursing H170607* [Educational Standards]. Retrieved from http://www.fldoe.org/academics/career-adult-edu/career-tech-edu/curriculum-frameworks/2018-19-frameworks/health-science.stml

Florida Department of Law Enforcement. (2017). *Drugs identified in deceased persons by Florida Medical Examiners* [Annual Report]. Retrieved from https://www.fdle.state.fl.us/MEC/Publications-and-Forms/Documents/Drugs-in-Deceased-Persons/2016-Annual-Drug-Report.aspx

Forster, P. L., Cavness, C., & Phelps, M. (1999, October). Staff training decreases use of seclusion and restraint in an acute psychiatric hospital. *Archives of Psychiatric Nursing*, *13*, 269-271.

Gacki-Smith, J., Juarez, A. M., Boyett, L., Homeyer, C., Robinson, L., & MacLean, S. L. (2009, July/August). Violence Against Nurses Working in US Emergency Departments. *Journal of Nursing Administration*, *39*, 340-349.

Gates, D. M., Gillespie, G. L., & Succop, P. (2011, March/April). Violence against nurses and its impact on stress and productivity. *Nursing Economics*, *29*, 59-66.

Gilbert, S. B. (2009, November 5). Psychiatric crash cart: Treatment strategies for the emergency room. *Advanced Emergency Nursing Journal, 31*, 298-308.

Gray, J. R., Grove, S. K., & Sutherland, S. (2017). *Burns and Grove's The Practice of Nursing Research; Appraisal, Synthesis, and Generation of Evidence* (8th ed.). St. Louis, Missouri: Elsevier.

Grindel, C. G. (2016, January-February). Clinical leadership: A call to action. *MEDSURG Nursing, 25*, 9-16.

Grindel, C. G. (2016, January/February). Clinical leadership: A call to action. *Med-Surg Nursing, 25*.

Gullich, I., Ramos, A. B., Anschau Zan, T. R., Scherer, C., & Mendoza-Sassi, R. A. (2013, September). Prevalence of anxiety in patients admitted to a university hospital in southern Brazil and associated factors. *Revista Brasileira de Epidemiologia, 16*, 644-657. http://dx.doi.org/http://dx.doi.org/10.1590/S1415-790X2013000300009

Gullich, I., Ramos, A. B., Anschau Zan, T. R., Scherer, C., & Mendoza-Sassi, R. A. (2013, September). Prevalence of anxiety in patients admitted to a university hospital in southern Brazil and associated factors. *Revista Brasileira de Epidemiologia, 16*, 644-657. http://dx.doi.org/http://dx.doi.org/10.1590/S1415-790X2013000300009

Harrington, C., Crider, M. C., Benner, P. E., & Malone, R. E. (2005). Advanced nursing training in health policy: Designing and implementin a new program. *Policy, Politics, & Nursing Practice, 6*, 99-108. http://dx.doi.org/10.1177/1527154405276070

Henson, B. (2010, November 4). Preventing interpersonal violence in emergency departments: Practical applications of criminology theory. *Violence and victims*, *25*, 553-565. Retrieved from https://search-proquest-com.ezp.waldenulibrary.org/docview/650828591?accountid=14872

Hodges, B. C., & Videto, D. M. (2011). *Assessment and Planning in Health Programs* (2 ed.). Sudbury, MA: Jones & Bartlett Learning.

Hogarth, K. M., Beattie, J., & Morphet, J. (2015, March 26). Nurses' attitutes towards the reporting of violence in the emergency department. *Australasian Emergency Nursing Journal*, *19*, 75-81. http://dx.doi.org/http://dx.doi.org/10.1016/j.aenj.2015.03.006

Institute for Healthcare Communication. (2011). Impact of communication in healthcare. Retrieved from https://healthcarecomm.org/about-us/impact-of-communication-in-healthcare/

Institute of Medicine. (2010). The future of nursing: Focus on education. Retrieved from http://www.nationalacademies.org/hmd/~/media/Files/Report%20Files/2010/The-Future-of-Nursing/Nursing%20Education%202010%20Brief.pdf

Izumi, S. (2013, October 1). Quality improvement in nursing: Administrative mandate or professional responsibilty? *Nursing Forum*, *47*, 260-267. http://dx.doi.org/10.1111/j.1744-6198.2012.00283.x

Jang, H., Song, Y., & Kang, H. (2017, September). Nurses' perception of patient safety culture and safety control in patient safety management activities. *Journal of Korean Academy of Nursing Administration*, *23*, 450-459. http://dx.doi.org/https://doi.org/10.11111/jkana.2017.23.4.450

Kennealy, P. J., Skeem, J. L., Manchak, S. M., & Louden, J. E. (2012). Firm, fair and caring officer-offender relationships protect against supervison failure. *Law and Human Behavior*, *36*, 496-505.

Kettner, P. M., Moroney, R. M., & Martin, L. L. (2017). *Designing and Managing Programs* (5th ed.). Los Angeles: Sage.

Kleissl-Muir, S., Raymond, A., & Rahman, M. A. (2018, October 15). Incidence and factors associated with substance abuse and patient-related violence in the emergency department: A literature review. *Australasian Emergency Care*, *21*, 159-170. http://dx.doi.org/https://doi.org/10.1016/j.auec.2018.10.004

Kvas, A., & Seljak, J. (2014, October 14). Sources of workplace violence against nurses. *Work*, *52*, 177-184.

Kvas, A., & Seljak, J. (2014, October 14). Sources of workplace violence against nurses. *Work*, *52*, 177-184. http://dx.doi.org/10.3233/WOR-152040

Laeeque, S. H., Bilal, A., Babar, S., Khan, Z., & Rahman, S. U. (2017, November 11). How patient-perpetrated workplace violence leads to turnover intention among nurses: The mediating mechanism of occupational stress and burnout. *Journal of Aggression, Maltreatment & Trauma, 27*, 96-118. http://dx.doi.org/https://doi.org/10.1080/10926771.2017.1410751

LaMorte, W. W. (2018). The social cognitive theory. Retrieved from http://sphweb.bumc.bu.edu/otlt/MPH-Modules/SB/BehavioralChangeTheories/BehavioralChangeTheories5.html

Lasater, K., Mood, L., Buchwach, D., & Dieckmann, N. F. (2015). Reducing incivility in the workplace: Results of a three-part educational intervention. *The Journal of Continuing Education in Nursing, 46*, 15-24.

Le, L. D., & Pharm, B. (2016, January 8). Healthcare facilities: Patient aggression/violence. *JBI Evidence Summary*, 1-5.

Lochead, T. (2009, September). Violence in the ED. *The Lamp*, 30-31. Retrieved from https://eds-a-ebscohost-com.ezp.waldenulibrary.org/eds/pdfviewer/pdfviewer?vid=1&sid=2454f578-1a57-41c2-829a-eb4fccab422d%40sdc-v-sessmgr01

Mason, V. M., Leslie, G., Lyons, P., Walke, E., & Griffin, M. (2014, July/August). Compassion fatigue, moral distress, and work engagement in surgical intensive care unit trauma nurses. *Dimensions of Critical Care Nursing*, 215-225. http://dx.doi.org/10.1097/DCC.0000000000000056

McClendon, S., Farbman, R., & Cipriano, P. F. (2018, April 18). ANA responds to the Joint Commission sentinel event alert on physical and verbal violence against health care workers. *Nursing World*.

McPhaul, K. M., London, M., & Lipscomb, J. A. (2013, January 31). A framework for translating workplace intervention research into evidence-based programs. *The Online Journal of Issues in Nursing, 18*.

Mealer, M., Burnham, E. L., Goode, C. J., Rothbaum, B., & Moss, M. (2009). The prevalence and impact of post traumatic stress disorder and burnout syndrome in nurses. Retrieved from https://www.ncbi.nlm.nih.gov/pmc/articles/PMC2919801/pdf/nihms211783.pdf

Montalvo, I. (2007, September 30). The National Database of Nursing Quality Indicators (NDNQI). *The Online Journal of Issues in Nursing, 12*. http://dx.doi.org/10.3912/OJIN.Vol12

National Association of State Mental Health Program Directors. (2006). *Six core strategies for reducing seclusion and restraint use* [Report]. Alexandria, VA: National Association of State Mental Health Program Directors.

Netsmart. (2018). EHR for medication-assisted addiction treatment. Retrieved from https://www.ntst.com/Communities-We-Serve/behavioral-health/medication-assisted-treatment/

Netsmart. (2018). The netsmart story. Retrieved from https://www.ntst.com/The-Netsmart-Story/

Nixon, W. B. (2018). New violence in the workplace fact sheet emphasizes prevention. Retrieved from https://www.securitymagazine.com/articles/83736-new-violence-in-the-workplace-fact-sheet-emphasizes-prevention

O'Hagan, M., Divis, M., & Long, J. (2008). *Best Practice in the reduction and elimination of seclusion and restraint - Seclusion: Time for change* [Educational standards]. Retrieved from https://www.mentalhealth.org.nz/assets/ResourceFinder/FINAL-SECLUSION-REDUCTION-BEST-PRACTICE-Research-Report.pdf

Occupational Safety and Health Administration. (2015). Workplace violence in healthcare; Understanding the challenge. Retrieved from https://www.osha.gov/Publications/OSHA3826.pdf

Occupational Safety and Health Administration. (n.d.). Workplace violence in healthcare; Understanding the challenge. Retrieved from https://www.osha.gov/Publications/OSHA3826.pdf

Office of Disease Prevention and Health Promotion. (2018). Soical determinants of health. Retrieved from https://www.healthypeople.gov/2020/topics-objectives/topic/social-determinants-of-health

Paterson, B., Miller, G., Bowie, V., & Ledbetter, D. (2008, May). Zero tolerance and violence in services for people with mental health needs. *Mental Health Practice, 11*, 26-31.

Phillips, J. P. (2016, April 28). Workplace violence against health care workers in the United States. *The New England Journal of Medicine*, 1661-1669. Retrieved from https://search-proquest-com.ezp.waldenulibrary.org/docview/1785294272/fulltextPDF/815C3293FB8B4720PQ/1?accountid=14872

Polk, L. V. (1997). Toward a middle-range theory of resilience. *Advances in Nursing Science*, *19*(3), 1-13. Retrieved from http://ovidsp.tx.ovid.com.ezp.waldenulibrary.org

Poremski, D., Woodhall-Melnik, J., Lemieux, A. J., & Stergiopoulos, V. (2016, February 1). Persisting barriers to employment for recently housed adults with mental illness who were homeless. *Journal of Urban Health: Bulletin of the New York Academy of Medicine*, *93*, 96-108. http://dx.doi.org/10.1007/s11524-015-0012-y

Rappleye, E. (2015). Average cost per inpatient day across 50 states. Retrieved from https://www.beckershospitalreview.com/finance/average-cost-per-inpatient-day-across-50-states.html

Rehfuess, E. A., Durao, S., Kyamanywa, P., Meerpohl, J. J., Young, T., & Rohwer, A. (2016). An approach for setting evidence-based and stakeholder-informed research priorities in low and middle income countries. *Bulletin of World Health Organization*, *94*, 297-305. http://dx.doi.org/http://dx.doi.org/10.2471/BLT.15.162966

Relias. (2018). Workplace violence. Retrieved from https://www.relias.com/resource/workplace-violence

Rodriguez-Acosta, R. L., Myers, D. J., Richardson, D. B., Lipscomb, H. J., Chen, J. C., & Dement, J. M. (2008, September 6). Physical assault among nursing staff employed in acute care. *Work*, *35*, 191-200.

Rosswurm, M., & Larrabee, J. H. (1999). A model for change to evidence-based practice. *Journal of Nursing Scholarship*, *31*, 317-348.

Sato, K., Wakabayashi, T., Kiyoshi-Teo, H., & Fukahori, H. (2012, December 16). Factors associated with nurses' reporting of patients' aggressive behavior: A cross-sectional survey. *International Journal of Nursing Studies*, *50*, 1368-1376. http://dx.doi.org/http://dx.doi.org/10.1016/j.ijnurstu.2012.12.011

Schmidt, M., & Haglund, K. (2017, September/October). Debrief in emergency departments to improve compassion fatique and promote resiliency. *Journal of Trauma Nursing*, *24*, 317-322. http://dx.doi.org/10.1097/JTN.0000000000000315

Sidhu, S., & Park, T. (2018, March 8). Nursing curriculum and bullying: An integrative literature review. *Nurse Education Today*, *65*, 169-176. http://dx.doi.org/https://doi.org/10.1016/j.nedt.2018.03.005

Snyder, L. A., Chen, P. Y., & Vacha-Haase, T. (2007). The underreporting gap in aggressive incidents from geriatric patients against certified nursing assistants. *Violence and Victims*, *22*, 367-379.

Sofield, L., & Salmond, S. W. (2003, July/August). Workplace violence: A focus on verbal abuse and intent to leave the organization. *Orthopaedic Nursing*, *22*, 274-283.

Speroni, K. G., Fitch, T., Dawson, E., Dugan, L., & Atherton, M. (2014, May). Incidence and cost of nurse workplace violence perpetrated by hospital patients or patient visitors. *Journal of Emergency Nursing, 40*, 218-228.

Stiver, K., Sharma, N., Geller, K., Smith, L., Stephens, J., Daoud, E., ... Mazzaferri, E. (2017). "Quiet at night": Reduced overnight vital sign monitoring linked to both safety and improvements in patients' perception of hospital sleep quality. *Patient Experience Journal, 4*, 90-96. Retrieved from https://pxjournal.org/cgi/viewcontent.cgi?article=1185&context=journal

Sublett, C. M. (2006, February). EBP: Pain control for prostate cancer patients receiving HDR brachytherapy. *Urologic Nursing, 26*, 63-66.

Substance Abuse and Mental Health Services Administrations. (2005). *Roadmap to seclusion and restraint free mental health services* [Educational standards]. Retrieved from Connecting Learners with Knowledge: https://www.clwk.ca/wp-content/uploads/buddyshared/SAMHSA-Roadmap-to-Seclusion-and-Restraint-Free-Mental-Health-Services.pdf

Suchy, K. (2010, July/August). A lack of standardization: The basis for the ethical issue surrounding quality and performance reports. *Jounral of Healthcare Management, 55*, 241-251.

Taylor, R. (2016, February 23). Nurses' perceptions of horizontal violence. *Global Qualitative Nursing Research, 3*, 1-9. http://dx.doi.org/10.1177/2333393616641002

Taylor, S. E. (1983, November). Adjustment to threatening events: A theory of cognitive adaptation. *American Psychologist*, 1161-1173.

The Joint Commission. (2018). Physical and verbal violence against health care workers. Retrieved from https://www.jointcommission.org/assets/1/18/SEA_59_Workplace_violence_4_13_18_FINAL.pdf

Trinkoff, A. M., Geiger-Brown, J. M., Caruso, C. C., Lipscomb, J. A., Johantgen, M., Nelson, A. L., ... Selby, V. L. (n.d.). Personal safety for nurses. *Patient Safety and Quality: An Evidence-Based Handbook for Nurses*, 1-36.

White, K. M., Dudley-Brown, S., & Terhaar, M. F. (2016). *Translation of evidence into nursing and health care* (2nd ed.). New York, NY: Springer Publishing Company, LLC.

Wienclaw, R. A. (2017). Communications in the workplace. *Salem Press Encyclopedia*. Retrieved from https://eds-b-ebscohost-com.ezp.waldenulibrary.org/eds/detail/detail?vid=7&sid=7989d38e-0765-4b54-83c8-ad594cb2b3a7%40pdc-v-sessmgr01&bdata=JnNpdGU9ZWRzLWxpdmUmc2NvcGU9c2l0ZQ%3d%3d#AN=89163589&db=ers

Zhao, S., Liu, H., Ma, H., Jiao, M., Li, Y., Hao, Y., ... Qiao, H. (2015, November 13). Coping with workplace violence in healthcare settings: Social support strategies. *International Journal of Environmental Research and Public Health*, *12*, 14429-14444. http://dx.doi.org/10.3390/ijerph21114429

Zysk, T. (2018, September/October). How to build resilience and reduce nurse burnout through better care team communication. *Health Management Technology*, 14-15. Retrieved from https://web-a-ebscohost-com.ezp.waldenulibrary.org/ehost/pdfviewer/pdfviewer?vid=3&sid=a3b14293-323c-4f41-8953-27345ecc2468%40sdc-v-sessmgr05

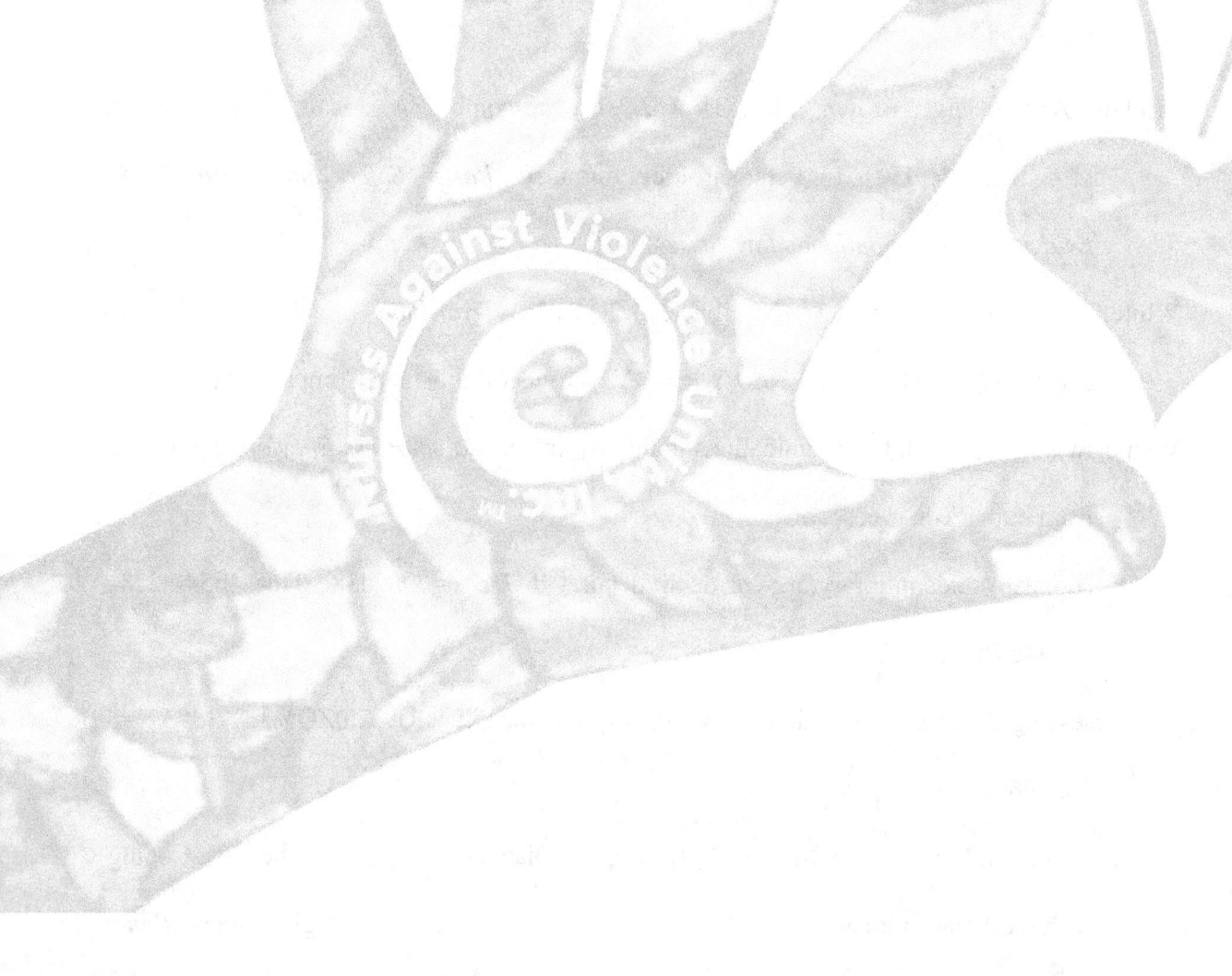

Book References

Advisory Board. (2016, May 3). Nearly 75 percent of all workplace assaults happen in health care, researchers find. *The Daily Briefing*.

American Association of Colleges of Nursing. (2006). The essentials of doctoral education for advanced nursing practice. Retrieved from http://www.aacn.nche.edu/dnp/Essentials.pdf

American Nurses Association. (2018, April 18). ANA responds to the Joint Commission sentinal event alert on physical and verbal violence against healthcare workers. *Nursing World*.

Angland, S., Dowling, M., & Casey, D. (2013, September 20). Nurses' perceptions of the factors which cause violence and aggression in the emergency department: A qualitative study. *International Emergency Nursing, 22*, 134-139. http://dx.doi.org/http://dx.doi.org/10.1016/j.ienj.2013.09.005

Armstrong, P. (2017). Bloom's Taxonomy. Retrieved from https://cft.vanderbilt.edu/guides-sub-pages/blooms-taxonomy/

Arnetz, J. E., Hamblin, L., Ager, J., Aranyos, D., Essenmacher, L., Upfal, M. J., & Luborsky, M. (2013, October 12). Using database reports to reduce workplace violence: Perceptions of hospital stakeholders. *Work, 51*, 51-59.

Arnetz, J. E., Hamblin, L., Ager, J., Luborsky, M., Upfal, M. J., Russell, J., & Essenmacher, L. (2015, May). Underreporting of Workplace Violence. *Workplace Health & Safety*, 200-210. http://dx.doi.org/10.1177/2165079915574684

Ashton, R. A., Morris, L., & Smith, I. (2017, December 20). A qualitative meta-synthesis of emergency department staff experiences of violence and aggression. *International Emergency Nursing*, *39*, 13-19. http://dx.doi.org/https://doi.org/10.1016/j.ienj.2017.12.004

Bandura, A. (1989, September). Human agency in social cognitive theory. *American Psychologist*, *44*, 1175-1184.

Bandura, A. (2001). Social cognitive theory: An agentic perspective. *Annual Review Psychology*, *52*, 1-26.

Bolvin, J. M. (2018, November). 2018 Nursing trends and salary results. *American Nurse Today*, *13*(11).

Bowman, S. (2013). Impact on electronic health record systems on information integrity: Quality and safety implications. Retrieved from https://www.ncbi.nlm.nih.gov/pmc/articles/PMC3797550/

Bureau of Labor Statistics. (2012, February). The recession of 2007-2009. *BLS spotlight on statistics*, 1-18. Retrieved from https://www.bls.gov/spotlight/2012/recession/pdf/recession_bls_spotlight.pdf

Center, D. (2018). Knowing oneself: The first step to be an effective member of an interprofessional team. *The Journal of Continuing Education in Nursing*, *49*, 397-399. http://dx.doi.org/10.3928/00220124-20180813-04

Chapman, R., Styles, I., Perry, L., & Combs, S. (2010). Nurses' experience of adjusting to workplace violence: A theory of adaptation. *International Journal of Mental Health Nursing, 19*, 186-194. http://dx.doi.org/10.1111/j.1447-0349.2009.00663.x

Chen, W., Huang, C., Hwang, J., & Chen, C. (2010, June 10). The relationship of health-related quality of life to workplace physical violence against nurses by psychiatric patients. *Quality of Life Research, 19*, 1155-1161. http://dx.doi.org/10.1007/s11136-010-9679-4

Colvin, & Sugai (1989). Stages of behavior escalation. Retrieved from https://k12engagement.unl.edu/Stages%20of%20Behavior%20Escalation.pdf

Communication 5: Effective listening and observation skills [Discussion comment]. (2018, March 12). Retrieved from https://www.nursingtimes.net/clinical-archive/assessment-skills/communication-5-effective-listening-and-observation-skills/7023622.article

Copeland, D., & Henry, M. (2017, April). Workplace violence and perceptions of safety among emergency department staff members: Experiences, expectations, tolerance, reporting, and recommendations. *Journal of Trauma Nursing, 24*, 65-77, E1-E2.

Cox, E. (2017, September 29). Violence in the health care workplace. *U.S. News & World Report*. Retrieved from https://health.usnews.com/health-care/for-better/articles/2017-09-29/violence-in-the-health-care-workplace

Dao Le, L., & Pharm, B. (2016, January 8). Healthcare facilities:Patient aggression/violence. *JBI Evidence Summary*. Retrieved from http://ovidsp.tx.ovid.com.ezp.waldenulibrary.org/sp-3.26.1a/ovidweb.cgi?&S=HABGFPNAHPDDMBLCNCGKMHDCOMHEAA00&Link+Set=S.sh.21%7c7%7csl_190

Davey, G. C. (2013). Mental health & Stigma. Retrieved from https://www.psychologytoday.com/us/blog/why-we-worry/201308/mental-health-stigma

de Carvalho, E. C., Oliveiro-Kumakura, A. R., & Vasconcelos Morais, S. C. (2016, April 12). Clinical reasoning in nursing: Teaching strategies and assessment tools. *Revista Brasileira de Enfermagem, 70*, 662-667. http://dx.doi.org/http://dx.doi.org/10.1590/0034-7167-2016-0509

DeMarco, M., & Tilson, E. R. (n.d.). Maslow in the classroom and the clinic. *Teaching Techniques, 70*, 91-94.

Department of Health & Human Services. (2017). Healthy People 2020. Retrieved from https://www.healthypeople.gov/sites/default/files/HP2020_brochure_with_LHI_508_FNL.pdf

Department of Mental Health Law & Policy. (2014). *Baker Act; The Florida Mental Health Act* [User reference guide]. Retrieved from http://www.dcf.state.fl.us/programs/samh/mentalhealth/laws/BakerActManual.pdf

Djulbegovic, B. (2014). A framework to bridge the gaps between evidence-based medicine, health outcomes, and improvement and implementation science. *Journal of Oncology Practice, 10*, 200-202.

Doody, C. M., & Doody, O. (2011, May). Introducing evidence into nursing practice: using the Iowa model. *British Journal of Nursing, 20*, 661-664.

Doran, D. M., Haynes, R. B., Kushniruk, A., Strauss, S., Grimshaw, J., McGillis-Hall, L., ... Jedras, D. (2010, September 30). Supporting evidence-based practice for nurses through information technologies. *Worldviews on Evidence-Based Nursing, 7*, 4-15.

DuBose, J. R., & Hadi, K. (2016, November 10). Improving inpatient environments to support patient sleep. *International Journal for Quality in Health Care, 28*, 540-553. http://dx.doi.org/https://doi.org/10.1093/intqhc/mzw079

Fasanya, B. K., & Dada, E. A. (2015, December 1). Workplace violence and safety issues in long-term medical care facilities: Nurses' perspectives. *Safety and Health at Work, 7*, 97-101.

Fawcett, J., & Garity, J. (2009). Chapter 1: Research and evidence-based nursing practice. *Evaluating Research for Evidence-Based Nursing*, 3-20.

Florida Department of Children and Families. (2014). Baker Act involuntary examination criteria, processes and timeframes. Retrieved from https://www.dcf.state.fl.us/programs/samh/MentalHealth/laws/bainvex.pdf

Florida Department of Education. (2018). *PSAV Programs; Practical Nursing H170607* [Educational Standards]. Retrieved from http://www.fldoe.org/academics/career-adult-edu/career-tech-edu/curriculum-frameworks/2018-19-frameworks/health-science.stml

Forsyth, D. M., Wright, T. L., Scherb, C. A., & Gaspar, P. M. (n.d.). Disseminating evidence-based practice projects: Poster design and evaluation. *Clinical Scholars Review, 3*, 14-21. http://dx.doi.org/10.1891/1939-2095.3.1.14

Gacki-Smith, J., Juarez, A. M., Boyett, L., Homeyer, C., Robinson, L., & MacLean, S. L. (2009, July/August). Violence Against Nurses Working in US Emergency Departments. *Journal of Nursing Administration, 39*, 340-349.

Gray, J. R., Grove, S. K., & Sutherland, S. (2017). *Burns and Grove's The Practice of Nursing Research; Appraisal, Synthesis, and Generation of Evidence* (8th ed.). St. Louis, Missouri: Elsevier.

Grindel, C. G. (2016, January-February). Clinical leadership: A call to action. *MEDSURG Nursing, 25*, 9-16.

Gullich, I., Ramos, A. B., Anschau Zan, T. R., Scherer, C., & Mendoza-Sassi, R. A. (2013, September). Prevalence of anxiety in patients admitted to a university hospital in southern Brazil and associated factors. *Revista Brasileira de Epidemiologia, 16*, 644-657. http://dx.doi.org/http://dx.doi.org/10.1590/S1415-790X2013000300009

Harrington, C., Crider, M. C., Benner, P. E., & Malone, R. E. (2005). Advanced nursing training in health policy: Designing and implementin a new program. *Policy, Politics, & Nursing Practice, 6*, 99-108. http://dx.doi.org/10.1177/1527154405276070

Henson, B. (2010, November 4). Preventing interpersonal violence in emergency departments: Practical applications of criminology theory. *Violence and victims, 25*, 553-565. Retrieved from https://search-proquest-com.ezp.waldenulibrary.org/docview/650828591?accountid=14872

Hodges, B. C., & Videto, D. M. (2011). *Assessment and Planning in Health Programs* (2 ed.). Sudbury, MA: Jones & Bartlett Learning.

Hogarth, K. M., Beattie, J., & Morphet, J. (2015, March 26). Nurses' attitutes towards the reporting of violence in the emergency department. *Australasian Emergency Nursing Journal*, *19*, 75-81. http://dx.doi.org/http://dx.doi.org/10.1016/j.aenj.2015.03.006

Homested, L. (2000, March). Institute of Medicine report: To Err is Human: Building a safer health care system. *The Florida Nurse*, *48*, 6. Retrieved from https://search-proquest-com.ezp.waldenulibrary.org/docview/230309579?accountid=14872

Huye, H. F., Connell, C. L., Cook, L. B., Yadrick, K., & Zoellner, J. (2014). Using the RE-AIM framework in formative evaluation and program planning for a nutrition intervention in the lower Mississippi delta. *Journal of Nutrition Education and Behavior*, *46*, 34-42.

Institute for Healthcare Communication. (2011). Impact of communication in healthcare. Retrieved from https://healthcarecomm.org/about-us/impact-of-communication-in-healthcare/

Institute of Medicine of the National Academies. (2010). *The future of nursing: Leading change, advancing health*. Retrieved from Institute of Medicine of the National Academies: https://web.archive.org/web/20150211165201/http://iom.edu/Reports/2010/The-Future-of-Nursing-Leading-Change-Advancing-Health.aspx

IOM Report, The Future of Nursing: Leading change, Advancing health: Milestones and challenges in expanding nursing science. (2011). Retrieved from https://class.waldenu.edu/bbcswebdav/institution/USW1/201930_27/DR_NURS/NURS_8500_WC/artifacts/USW1_NURS_8500_IOMReport_Bleich.pdf

Izumi, S. (2013, October 1). Quality improvement in nursing: Administrative mandate or professional responsibilty? *Nursing Forum*, *47*, 260-267. http://dx.doi.org/10.1111/j.1744-6198.2012.00283.x

Jaruzel, C. B., & Gregoski, M. J. (2017, February). Instruments to measure preoperative acute situational anxiety: An integrative view. *American Association of Nurse Anesthetists*, *85*, 31-35.

Kennealy, P. J., Skeem, J. L., Manchak, S. M., & Louden, J. E. (2012). Firm, fair and caring officer-offender relationships protect against supervison failure. *Law and Human Behavior*, *36*, 496-505.

Kettner, P. M., Moroney, R. M., & Martin, L. L. (2017). *Designing and Managing Programs* (5th ed.). Los Angeles: Sage.

Kondo, K. K., Damberg, C. L., Mendelson, A., Motu'apuaka, M., Freeman, M., O'Neil, M., ... Kansagara, D. (2016, March 7). Implementation processes and pay for performance in healthcare: A systematic review. *JGIM: Journal Of General Internal Medicine*, *31*, S61-9. http://dx.doi.org/10.1007/s11606-015-3567-0

Laeeque, S. H., Bilal, A., Babar, S., Khan, Z., & Rahman, S. U. (2017, November 11). How patient-perpetrated workplace violence leads to turnover intention among nurses: The mediating mechanism of occupational stress and burnout. *Journal of Aggression, Maltreatment & Trauma*, *27*, 96-118. http://dx.doi.org/https://doi.org/10.1080/10926771.2017.1410751

Lasater, K., Mood, L., Buchwach, D., & Dieckmann, N. F. (2015). Reducing incivility in the workplace: Results of a three-part educational intervention. *The Journal of Continuing Education in Nursing*, *46*, 15-24.

Lee, J., Lee, Y. J., Bae, J., & Seo, M. (2016, August 9). Registered nurses' clinical reasoning skills and reasoning process: A think-aloud study. *Nurse Education Today*, *46*, 75-80.

Martin, R. E., Adamson, S., Korchinski, M., Granger-Brown, A., Ramsden, V. R., Buxton, J. A., ... Hislop, T. G. (2013). Incarcerated women develop a nutrition and fitness program: Participatory research. *International Journal of Prisoner Health*, *9*, 142-150. http://dx.doi.org/10.1108/IJPH-03-2013-0015

Mason, V. M., Leslie, G., Lyons, P., Walke, E., & Griffin, M. (2014, July/August). Compassion fatigue, moral distress, and work engagement in surgical intensive care unit trauma nurses. *Dimensions of Critical Care Nursing*, 215-225. http://dx.doi.org/10.1097/DCC.0000000000000056

McClendon, S., Farbman, R., & Cipriano, P. F. (2018, April 18). ANA responds to the Joint Commission sentinel event alert on physical and verbal violence against health care workers. *Nursing World*.

McEwen, M., & Wills, E. M. (2014). *Theoretical Basis for Nursing* (4th ed.). Philadelphia: Wolters Kluwer.

McPhaul, K. M., London, M., & Lipscomb, J. A. (2013, January 31). A framework for translating workplace intervention research into evidence-based programs. *The Online Journal of Issues in Nursing*, *18*.

Mealer, M., Burnham, E. L., Goode, C. J., Rothbaum, B., & Moss, M. (2009). The prevalence and impact of post traumatic stress disorder and burnout syndrome in nurses. Retrieved from https://www.ncbi.nlm.nih.gov/pmc/articles/PMC2919801/pdf/nihms211783.pdf

Montalvo, I. (2007). *American Nurses Association nursing sensitive measures National Database of Nursing Quality Indicators (NDNQI)* [PowerPoint slides]. Retrieved from https://www.ncvhs.hhs.gov/wp-content/uploads/2014/05/070619p8.pdf

Moran, K., Burson, R., & Conrad, D. (2017). *The Doctor of Nursing Practice Scholarly Project: A Framework for Success* (2nd ed.). Burlington, MA: Jones & Bartlett Learning.

National Institute of Mental Health. (2017). Mental Illness - Statistics. Retrieved from https://www.nimh.nih.gov/health/statistics/mental-illness.shtml

Nearly 75 percent of all workplace assaults happen in health care, researchers find. (2016). Retrieved from https://www.advisory.com/daily-briefing/2016/05/03/nearly-75-percent-of-all-workplace-assaults-happen-in-health-care

Nurse Practice Act, XXXII Florida Statute §§ 464.018 (1m) (2018).

Occupational Safety and Health Administration. (2015). Workplace violence in healthcare; Understanding the challenge. Retrieved from https://www.osha.gov/Publications/OSHA3826.pdf

Occupational Safety and Health Administration. (n.d.). Workplace violence in healthcare; Understanding the challenge. Retrieved from https://www.osha.gov/Publications/OSHA3826.pdf

Office of Disease Prevention and Health Promotion. (2018). Mental health and mental disorders. Retrieved from https://www.healthypeople.gov/2020/topics-objectives/topic/mental-health-and-mental-disorders

Office of Disease Prevention and Health Promotion. (2018). Mental health and mental disorders. Retrieved from https://www.healthypeople.gov/2020/topics-objectives/topic/mental-health-and-mental-disorders

Paterson, B., Miller, G., Bowie, V., & Ledbetter, D. (2008, May). Zero tolerance and violence in services for people with mental health needs. *Mental Health Practice, 11*, 26-31.

Phillips, J. P. (2016, April 28). Workplace violence against health care workers in the United States. *The New England Journal of Medicine*, 1661-1669. Retrieved from https://search-proquest-com.ezp.waldenulibrary.org/docview/1785294272/fulltextPDF/815C3293FB8B4720PQ/1?accountid=14872

Polk, L. V. (1997). Toward a middle-range theory of resilience. *Advances in Nursing Science, 19*(3), 1-13. Retrieved from http://ovidsp.tx.ovid.com.ezp.waldenulibrary.org

Poremski, D., Woodhall-Melnik, J., Lemieux, A. J., & Stergiopoulos, V. (2016, February 1). Persisting barriers to employment for recently housed adults with mental illness who were homeless. *Journal of Urban Health: Bulletin of the New York Academy of Medicine, 93*, 96-108. http://dx.doi.org/10.1007/s11524-015-0012-y

Rappleye, E. (2015). Average cost per inpatient day across 50 states. Retrieved from https://www.beckershospitalreview.com/finance/average-cost-per-inpatient-day-across-50-states.html

Rehfuess, E. A., Durao, S., Kyamanywa, P., Meerpohl, J. J., Young, T., & Rohwer, A. (2016). An approach for setting evidence-based and stakeholder-informed research priorities in low and middle income countries. *Bulletin of World Health Organization, 94*, 297-305. http://dx.doi.org/http://dx.doi.org/10.2471/BLT.15.162966

Ribeiro, V. F., Filho, C. F., Valenti, V. E., Ferreira, M., Abreu, L. D., Carvalho, T. D., ... Ferreira, C. (2014, May 9). Prevalence of burn-out syndrome in clinical nurses at a hospital of excellence. *International Archives of Medicine, 7*(22). http://dx.doi.org/10.1186/1755-7682-7-22

Rosswurm, M., & Larrabee, J. H. (1999). A model for change to evidence-based practice. *Journal of Nursing Scholarship, 31*, 317-348.

Schmidt, M., & Haglund, K. (2017, September/October). Debrief in emergency departments to improve compassion fatique and promote resiliency. *Journal of Trauma Nursing, 24*, 317-322. http://dx.doi.org/10.1097/JTN.0000000000000315

Simmons, B. (2009, December 4). Clinical reasoning: Concept analysis. *Journal of Advanced Nursing, 66*, 1151-1158.

Sofield, L., & Salmond, S. W. (2003, July/August). Workplace violence: A focus on verbal abuse and intent to leave the organization. *Orthopaedic Nursing, 22*, 274-283.

Speroni, K. G., Fitch, T., Dawson, E., Dugan, L., & Atherton, M. (2014, May). Incidence and cost of nurse workplace violence perpetrated by hospital patients or patient visitors. *Journal of Emergency Nursing, 40*, 218-228.

Sublett, C. M. (2006, February). EBP: Pain control for prostate cancer patients receiving HDR brachytherapy. *Urologic Nursing, 26*, 63-66.

Substance Abuse and Mental Health Services Administration. (2018). Prevention of substance abuse and mental illness. Retrieved from https://www.samhsa.gov/prevention

Suchy, K. (2010, July/August). A lack of standardization: The basis for the ethical issue surrounding quality and performance reports. *Jounral of Healthcare Management, 55*, 241-251.

Taylor, R. (2016, February 23). Nurses' perceptions of horizontal violence. *Global Qualitative Nursing Research, 3*, 1-9. http://dx.doi.org/10.1177/2333393616641002

Terry, A. J. (2018). *Clinical Research for the Doctor of Nursing Practice* (3rd ed.). Burlington, MA: Jones & Bartlett Learning.

The Joint Commission. (2018). Physical and verbal violence against health care workers. Retrieved from https://www.jointcommission.org/assets/1/18/SEA_59_Workplace_violence_4_13_18_FINAL.pdf

The Office of the National Coordinator for Health Information Technology. (2017). *Connecting public health information systems and health information exchange organizations* [Report]. Retrieved from https://www.healthit.gov/sites/default/files/FINAL_ONC_PH_HIE_090122017.pdf

Trinkoff, A. M., Geiger-Brown, J. M., Caruso, C. C., Lipscomb, J. A., Johantgen, M., Nelson, A. L., ... Selby, V. L. (n.d.). Personal safety for nurses. *Patient Safety and Quality: An Evidence-Based Handbook for Nurses*, 1-36.

White, K. M., Dudley-Brown, S., & Terhaar, M. F. (2016). *Translation of evidence into nursing and health care* (2nd ed.). New York, NY: Springer Publishing Company, LLC.

Wienclaw, R. A. (2017). Communications in the workplace. *Salem Press Encylopedia*. Retrieved from https://eds-b-ebscohost-com.ezp.waldenulibrary.org/eds/detail/detail?vid=7&sid=7989d38e-0765-4b54-83c8-ad594cb2b3a7%40pdc-v-sessmgr01&bdata=JnNpdGU9ZWRzLWxpdmUmc2NvcGU9c2l0ZQ%3d%3d#AN=89163589&db=ers

Yusof, M., & Sahroni, M. N. (2018, March 27). Investigating health information systems-induced errors. *International Journal of Health Care Quality Assurance*, *31*, 1014-1029. http://dx.doi.org/10.1108/IJHCQA-07-2017-0125

Zhao, S., Liu, H., Ma, H., Jiao, M., Li, Y., Hao, Y., ... Qiao, H. (2015, November 13). Coping with workplace violence in healthcare settings: Social support strategies. *International Journal of Environmental Research and Public Health*, *12*, 14429-14444. http://dx.doi.org/10.3390/ijerph21114429

Zysk, T. (2018, September/October). How to build resilience and reduce nurse burnout through better care team communication. *Health Management Technology*, 14-15. Retrieved from https://web-a-ebscohost-com.ezp.waldenulibrary.org/ehost/pdfviewer/pdfviewer?vid=3&sid=a3b14293-323c-4f41-8953-27345ecc2468%40sdc-v-sessmgr05

Thank you for taking the time to read a portion of what has gone into this DNP project and the other that drives the Nurses Against Violence Unite, Inc. mission. We love our jobs; we love what we do. It is a matter of human needs, safety and being heard when something is not working, we want to help employers to make it better…we are the frontline of healthcare, the organizational bottom-line. When in reality, we should not be regarded as such. We see what you do not. Our motivation is to be the best we can be for our patients, families and to feel rewarded emotionally by doing what we know and love, this is why we went to school and worked so hard to be a nurse. Our motivation is to keep the human in healthcare, for the best interest to heal a nation and ourselves. ~Dr. Sandy

www.ingramcontent.com/pod-product-compliance
Lightning Source LLC
Chambersburg PA
CBHW080455220526
45465CB00006B/2280